PRACTICAL GUIDE SERIES

CDT 2019 Coding Companion

Help Guide for the Dental Team

ADA American Dental Association®

America's leading advocate for oral health

Acknowledgements

The ADA would like to acknowledge contributions made by the following individuals to this publication, in addition to the chapter authors:

Editorial Panel – Council on Dental Benefit Programs' Subcommittee on Coding and Transactions

Dr. Thomas a'Becket; Dr. Christopher Bulnes; Dr. James Hollingsworth; Dr. Martin Makowski; Dr. Randall Markarian; Dr. Mark Mihalo; Dr. Cynthia Olenwine; and Dr. Steven Snyder

ADA Practice Institute – Center for Dental Benefits, Coding and Quality

Dr. Krishna Avaramudhan, Senior Director; Frank Pokorny, MBA, Senior Manager; and Stacy Starnes, Dental Codes Advisor

ADA Department of Product Development and Sales

Kathy Pulkrabek, Manager/Editor, Professional Products and Carolyn Tatar, MBA, Senior Manager, Product Development

We also want to acknowledge the permissions to reprint:

- Artwork provided by Glidewell Laboratories used in the discussion of Implant procedures, which are captioned: *"Image courtesy of Glidewell Laboratories."*
- The ADA publication *A Guide to Reporting D4346* (©2018 American Dental Association) in Appendix 2.
- The ADA publication *ADA Guide to Dental Procedures Reported with Area of the Oral Cavity or Tooth Anatomy (or Both)* (©2018 American Dental Association) in Appendix 2.

To order the current edition of this publication, please visit the American Dental Association's online catalog at adacatalog.org or call 1.800.947.4746.

CDT 2019 Coding Companion

Table of Contents

Section 3. Appendices

Section 1.

The CDT Code: What It Is and How To Use It

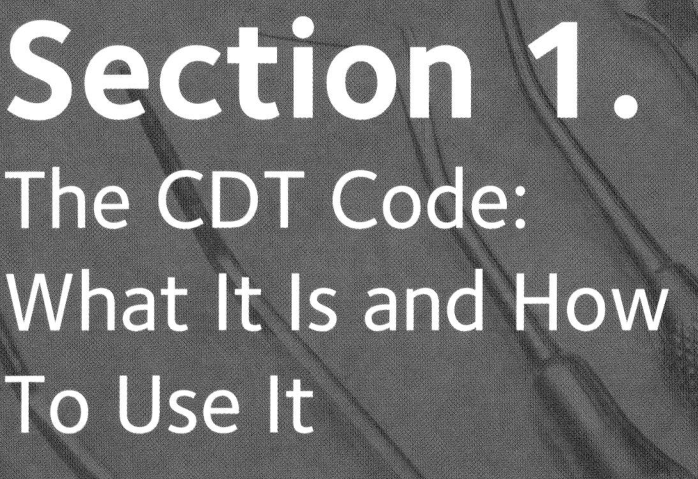

Section 1
The CDT Code: What It Is and How to Use It

A Brief History

The CDT Code was first published in 1969 as the "Uniform Code on Dental Procedures and Nomenclature" in the Journal of the American Dental Association. It originally consisted of numbers and a brief name, or nomenclature. Since 1990, the CDT Code has been published in the American Dental Association's dental reference manual titled Current Dental Terminology (CDT). The CDT Code version published in CDT-1 (1990) was marked by the addition of descriptors (a written narrative that provides further definition and the intended use of a dental procedure code) for most of the procedure codes.

The American Dental Association is the copyright owner and publisher of the CDT Code. New versions are published every year and become effective January 1st.

Federal regulations and legislation arising from the Health Insurance Portability and Accountability Act of 1996 (HIPAA) require all payers to accept HIPAA standard electronic dental claim. One data element on the electronic dental claim is the dental procedure code, which must be from the CDT Code – specifically the version that is in effect on the date of service.

Purpose

The CDT Code supports uniform, consistent, and accurate documentation of services delivered. This information is used in several ways:

- To provide for the efficient processing of dental claims
- To populate an electronic health record
- To record services to be delivered in a treatment plan

Note: Treatment plans must be developed according to professional standards, not according to provisions of the dental benefit contract. Always keep in mind that the existence of a procedure code does not guarantee that the procedure is a covered service.

Categories of Service

The CDT Code is organized into twelve categories of service, each with its own series of five-digit alphanumeric codes. These categories:

- Exist solely as a means to organize the CDT Code
- Reflect dental services that are considered similar in purpose
- Contain CDT codes that are available to document services delivered by anyone acting within the scope of their state law (for example, a dentist in general practice uses D7140 that is found in the oral and maxillofacial surgery category to document an extraction).

#	Name	Code Range	Description in commonly used terms*
I.	Diagnostic	D0100-D0999	Examinations, X-rays, pathology lab procedures
II.	Preventive	D1000-D1999	Cleanings (prophy), fluoride, sealants
III.	Restorative	D2000-D2999	Fillings, crowns and other related procedures
IV.	Endodontics	D3000-D3999	Root canals
V.	Periodontics	D4000-D4999	Surgical and non-surgical treatments of the gums and tooth supporting bone
VI.	Prosthodontics – removable	D5000-D5899	Dentures – partials and "flippers"
VII.	Maxillofacial Prosthetics	D5900-D5999	Facial, ocular and various other prostheses.
VIII.	Implant Services	D6000-D6199	Implants and implant restorations
IX.	Prosthodontics – fixed	D6200-D6999	Cemented bridges
X.	Oral & Maxillofacial Surgery	D7000-D7999	Extractions, surgical procedures, biopsies, treatment of fractures and injuries
XI.	Orthodontics	D8000-D8999	Braces
XII.	Adjunctive General Services	D9000-D9999	Miscellaneous services including anesthesia, professional visits, therapeutic drugs, bleaching, occlusal adjustment

* The language used in the "Description" column has been simplified using common non-clinical terms. It is not technical terminology.

Subcategories

All CDT Code categories of service are subdivided into one or more subcategories to aid navigation through the code set. For example, subcategories in the Diagnostic category of service include:

- Clinical Oral Evaluations
- Diagnostic Imaging
- Tests and Examinations

Note: CDT Code entries are *not always* in numerical order within a category of service. As the CDT Code grows and evolves, there are times when there is no sequential number available for a new entry that is related to an existing code.

Components of a CDT Code Entry

Every dental procedure code within a category of service has at least the first two and sometimes all three of the following components:

Procedure Code – A five-character alphanumeric code beginning with the letter "D" that identifies a specific dental procedure. Each procedure code is printed in **boldface type** in the CDT manual and cannot be changed or abbreviated.

Dental Procedure Code – five character alphanumeric beginning with "D"

sealant – per tooth
Mechanically and/or chemically prepared enamel surface sealed to prevent decay

Nomenclature – The written, literal definition of a procedure code. Each code has a nomenclature that is printed in **boldface** type in the CDT manual. Nomenclature may be abbreviated only when printed on claim forms or other documents that are subject to space limitation. Any such abbreviation does not constitute a change to the nomenclature.

Nomenclature (name) – written title of the procedure

D1351 **sealant – per tooth**
Mechanically and/or chemically prepared enamel surface sealed to prevent decay

Descriptor – A written narrative that provides further definition and describes the intended use of a dental procedure code. A descriptor is not provided for every procedure code. Descriptors that apply to a series of procedure codes may precede that series of codes; otherwise a descriptor will follow the applicable procedure code and its nomenclature. When present, descriptors are printed in regular typeface in the CDT manual. Descriptors as published cannot be added, abbreviated or otherwise changed.

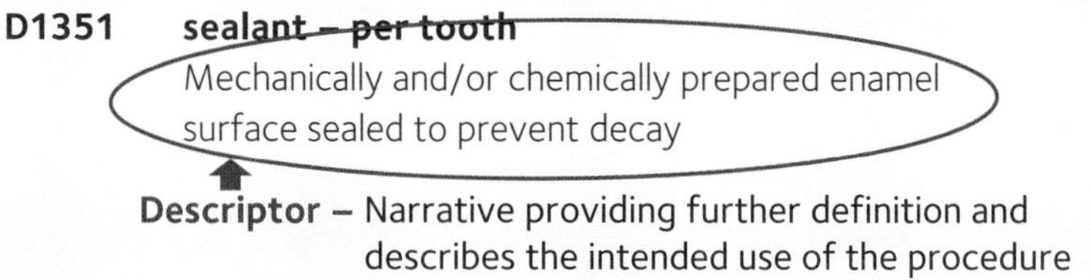
D1351
sealant – per tooth
Mechanically and/or chemically prepared enamel surface sealed to prevent decay
Descriptor – Narrative providing further definition and describes the intended use of the procedure

Descriptors are a very important component. Understanding the descriptor can help determine whether the procedure code accurately describes the service provided to a patient. This information can also help resolve questions about the accuracy of claim submissions.

Note: Your practice management software may not include entire CDT Code entries as some, due to space limitations, truncate nomenclatures and omit descriptors. With the current CDT Manual at hand you will have the complete entries for all CDT codes, which will help you select the appropriate code to document and report the service delivered.

What If There is No Code Describing a Procedure?

The complete CDT Code entry, described above, published in the current CDT Manual is used to determine the procedure code for documenting and reporting a service provided to a patient. But, what if there is no CDT code that, in the dentist's opinion, is applicable to the service? The available and appropriate option is to use an "unspecified procedure, by report" code, also known as a "999" code. These codes (e.g., **D2999 unspecified restorative procedure, by report**) are in every category of service, and when used must include a supporting narrative that explains the service provided.

A third-party payer may request additional documentation of certain procedures regardless of the presence of the narrative. Note, too, that dental benefit plan coverage limitations and exclusions, and where applicable the provisions of a participating provider agreement, affect third-party payer claim adjudication and reimbursement.

Narratives for "By Report" Codes

There are two types of CDT codes that require an explanatory narrative. The first and most readily known type are the "unspecified...procedure, by report" codes found in every category of service. Second are those codes in several categories that include "by report" in their nomenclatures – as seen in the following two examples.

D5862 precision attachment, by report
Each set of male and female components should be reported as one precision attachment. Describe the type of attachment used.

D6100 implant removal, by report
This procedure involves the surgical removal of an implant. Describe procedure.

When preparing a narrative report, first try and put yourself in the claim examiner's position. Your goal is to describe what you did and why, in a writing style and tone of an explanation to a friendly colleague. A good report is a clear and concise narrative that includes, as needed:

- Clinical condition of the oral cavity
- Description of the procedure performed
- Specific reasons why the procedure was needed, or extra time or material was needed
- How new technology enabled delivery
- Specific information required by a participating provider contract

Both the ADA Dental Claim Form and the HIPAA standard electronic dental claim transaction support transmittal of your narrative. If the "Remarks" field on the paper form does not provide enough space for you to say what you need to say, additional sheets may be included. Check with your practice management system vendor to learn how a narrative is included on your electronic claim submission.

Clarity is crucial. Do not assume that the reader will be familiar with acronyms or abbreviations you use on your patient records. Be sure to proofread the text before inclusion with the claim submission.

What do you think of this "by report" narrative?

> 1/2 carp anestetic 4% w/10.5 epinephrine administered. Explained procedure with patient's mother. Laser gingivectomy #8&9 and frenulectomy for max ant. Patient tolerated procedure well. Coagulation observed. Removed 2 mm of hyperplastic gingival #8 and 1.5 mm on #9 in facial and contured interseptal region. Raised max labial attendant 5 mm. Coagulation observed. POIG. Patient given rinse and cold sore meds for topical anesthisia.

It is a real-life example – shown exactly as submitted – that looks more like quickly written notes from the patient's record, with acronyms, misspellings and abbreviations that may confuse the reader. The entire claim was returned unprocessed.

Acronyms, abbreviations, and misspelled words hinder understanding. Narrative templates should be avoided, but if used the dentist remains obligated to review and approve the completed work before submission.

Now let's look at how the returned report narrative might have looked if written clearly.

> Patient age 5 presented with hyperplastic gingival tissue, and short and taut lingual frenum. Parent stated that child suffered from Aichmophobia, which could be diminished by anesthesia and use of laser in lieu of scalpel.
>
> Administered 1/2 carpule 4% Citanest Forte DENTAL with epinephrine. Used laser to: 1) remove 2 mm of hyperplastic gingival tissue from #8 and 1.5 mm on #9; 2) excise lingual frenum; and 3) cauterize wound. Coagulation was observed.
>
> Patient received post-operative instructions, oral antibiotic (amoxicillin) and oral analgesic (benzocaine) before release. Procedures delivered were: D4211 (gingivectomy or gingivoplasty); D7960 (frenulectomy); D9215 (local anesthesia); D9630 (drugs dispensed for home use).

This is a clear and concise report that answers the "what and why" questions the claims reviewer will be asking. It establishes clinical need and the procedure's positive outcome as expected.

CDT Code Maintenance: Additions, Revisions and Deletions

The ADA's Council on Dental Benefit Programs (CDBP) is responsible for CDT Code maintenance. In 2012, it established its Code Maintenance Committee (CMC), which convenes annually to vote on CDT Code action requests. Accepted requests are incorporated into the next version, which is effective on January 1st yearly.

Features of the maintenance process now in place are:

1. The CMC, a 21-member body comprised of representatives from numerous sectors of the dental community (such as third-party payers and dental specialties, including public health dentistry), that votes to accept, amend or decline a CDT Code action request.
2. A summary of action requests to be addressed at each CMC meeting is posted for download on ***ADA.org/cdt***, including information on how to obtain a copy of the complete request form.
3. During a CMC meeting the chair encourages submitters of action requests and any other interested party to voice their comments on any requests to the committee's members.
4. During a CMC meeting the committee members discuss action requests and cast their votes.
5. The ADA Council on Dental Benefit Programs sends notices of action taken to each person or entity that submitted a CDT Code action request and posts the results on ***ADA.org/cdt***.

Please visit the ADA's web page ***ADA.org/cdt*** for more information.

The CDT Code changes for many reasons, including technology or materials that have led to new procedures not currently in the taxonomy, or the need to improve clarity and accuracy of nomenclature and descriptors. Anyone may submit an action request.

For further assistance please contact the ADA Member Service Center at 312.440.2500.

Dental Procedure Codes (CDT) and Diagnosis Codes (ICD)

Dentists, through education and experience, diagnose a patient's oral health prior to treatment plan preparation and delivery of necessary dental services. However, for diagnoses, codified clinical documentation or reporting on a dental claim is not a routine activity. Change is afoot and your colleagues on the ADA Council on Dental Benefit Programs offer a look ahead to help you prepare for documenting and reporting diagnosis codes if and when required.

Both the ADA Dental Claim Form and the HIPAA standard electronic dental claim transaction are able to report up to four diagnosis codes. This capability was added to the claim forms with the expectation that ICD (International Classification of Diseases) would, at some point, become a required data element for dental claim adjudication.

Why should dentists be concerned with ICD codes when the ADA has developed SNODENT?

SNODENT is a clinical terminology designed for use with electronic health records, and it differs from ICD in three ways:

1. It is an input code set.
2. It has broader scope and specificity.
3. It may be mapped to ICD as needed on a dental claim.

Federal regulations published under the auspices of HIPAA's Administrative Simplification provisions specify only ICD codes as valid on claim submissions.

Most – but not all – diagnoses will be reported using an entry from the "Diseases of Oral Cavity" in ICD-10-CM (K00 – K14 series). ICD-10-CM became the HIPAA standard on October 1, 2015. It is a code set maintained by federal government agencies and available online at *www.cms.gov/Medicare/Coding/ICD10*.

Dentists and their staff are urged to familiarize themselves with the particulars of patients' dental benefits plans claim preparation and submission requirements. In addition, pay close attention to communications from dental plans regarding additional benefits for services connected to systemic health or about dental plans' intentions to require diagnostic codes on dental claim submissions.

Note: There is no immediate and universal mandate to include an ICD-10-CM code on all dental claims. We also emphasize that dental benefit plans are unlikely to establish identical diagnostic code reporting requirements in the foreseeable future. You should check with each plan for its requirements.

Section 3 contains the appendix titled "CDT Code to ICD (Diagnosis) Code Cross-Walk," an aid to recordkeeping and claim preparation. Tables in this appendix link frequently reported CDT codes with one or more possible ICD-10-CM diagnostic codes. Please note that these tables are not all inclusive but do serve as a guide for commonly occurring conditions.

Note: Several chapters in Section 2 include additional information on ICD-10-CM codes pertinent to the procedures listed in the CDT Code's category of service.

Dentists, by virtue of their clinical education, experience, and professional ethics, are the individuals responsible for diagnosis. As such, a dentist is also obligated to select the appropriate diagnosis code for patient records and claim submission. It is quite possible that other diagnoses and their associated codes may be appropriate for a given clinical scenario.

As you study these tables please note:

1. Some address a single CDT code (e.g., preventive resin restoration), and others include a suite of related procedure codes (e.g., resin-based composite).
2. Likewise, the number of suggested ICD-10-CM diagnosis codes in a table can range from one (e.g., gingival recession for eight graft codes) to more than 10.
3. Several contain suggested diagnosis codes that are not from the "Diseases of the Oral Cavity" section ICD-10-CM; there are circumstances (e.g., vehicle accidents, workers compensation) where other sections of the ICD code set has pertinent entries.
4. Most of the frequently cited ICD codes applicable to dental procedures are found in the Kxx series (Diseases of oral cavity and salivary glands), and to a lesser degree from three other series — Rxx (Symptoms, signs and abnormal clinical and laboratory findings); Sxx (Injury, poisoning and certain other consequences of external causes); and Zxx (Factors influencing health status and contact with health services).
5. Some ICD code terms contain words that are not commonly used in the US. These words, identified by an asterisk (*), are defined in the ADA online glossary: *ADA.org/en/publications/cdt/glossary-of-dental-clinical-and-administrative-ter*

Similar CDT to ICD tables are posted in the ADA's Center for Professional Success (CPS) website at ***success.ada.org/en/dental-benefits/icd-and-cdt-codes***.

These online tables may be updated more frequently than those in print as changes to ICD-10-CM occur on a schedule that differs from the CDT Code's timetable.

Dental Procedure Codes vs. Medical Procedure Codes

The CDT Code is the source for procedure codes used when submitting claims to dental benefit plans on either the ADA Dental Claim Form or the HIPAA standard electronic dental claim transaction. There may be times when a dentist's services are submitted to a patient's medical benefit plan. When this happens, not only is there a different claim form, but there are also different procedure codes that must be used. None of these are developed or maintained by the ADA.

Filing claims with a patient's medical benefit plan can be done using the "1500" paper form or HIPAA electronic equivalent. Information on the 1500 Claim Form, including completion instructions, can be found at the American Medical Association's (AMA) National Uniform Claim Committee website *www.nucc.org*.

Medical procedure codes come from two sources, the AMA's Current Procedure Terminology (CPT) code set and the federal government's Healthcare Common Procedure Code Set (HCPCS). All medical diagnosis codes come from the federal government's International Classification of Diseases-10th Revision-Clinical Modification (ICD-10-CM) code set.

Note: When selecting a medical procedure code, the rule of thumb is to first look at the CPT code set to determine if there is an appropriate code to use. If there is none, a HCPCS code may be used.

Sources for medical procedure codes include, but are not limited to:

1. American Medical Association
   https://commerce.ama-assn.org/store
   800.621.8335

2. Centers for Medicare and Medicaid Services (HCPCS)
   www.cms.hhs.gov/HCPCSReleaseCodeSets

Sources for ICD-10-CM diagnosis codes include, but are not limited to:

1. National Center for Health Statistics
   https://www.cdc.gov/nchs/icd/index.htm

2. ADA Catalog
   Diagnostic Coding for Dental Claim Submission by Charles Blair, D.D.S.
   ADAcatalog.org
   800.947.4746

3. PMIC Coding and Compliance
   http://icd10coding.com

One source of dental to medical procedure cross coding information is:

- ADA Catalog
  Medical-Dental Cross Coding with Confidence by Charles Blair, D.D.S.
  ADAcatalog.org
  800.947.4746

Claim Rejection: Payer Misuse of the CDT Code or Something Else?

Some claims will be rejected by a third-party payer and the reason for denial helps determine what should be done next. "The existence of a dental procedure code does not mean that the procedure is a covered or reimbursed benefit," is a quote from the preface of the first (1990) and every later edition of the CDT manual. This is an important concept as available coverage is determined by dental benefit plan design. Plan limitations and exclusions vary, which means a procedure that is covered by one patient's benefit plan may not be covered by another patient's plan.

In August 2000, HIPAA (Health Insurance Portability and Accountability Act of 1996) Subtitle F (Administrative Simplification) regulations named the Code on Dental Procedures and Nomenclature (CDT Code) as the federal standard for reporting dental procedures on electronic dental claims. Some have interpreted this to mean that since the CDT Code is a national standard, payers must provide reimbursement for any valid procedure code reported on a claim. This is an erroneous interpretation as the HIPAA regulations are limited to four statements:

1. A standard electronic dental claim may only contain procedures found in the CDT Code.
2. A dentist must submit the procedure code that is valid on the date of service.
3. A payer may not refuse to accept for processing a claim with a valid procedure code.
4. A payer's benefit plan design and adjudication policies apply when processing a claim.

In other words, HIPAA establishes a standard for communicating information about services provided to a patient. HIPAA does not influence a payer's claim adjudication process (e.g., application of policies and benefit limitations and exclusions).

An explanation of benefits that shows reimbursement for fewer services or for different procedure codes than reported on the claim raises eyebrows and prompts dentists to call the ADA and ask, "How can this happen? Isn't the third-party payer doing something wrong or illegal? It looks like the CDT Code is being misused." The first step in answering these questions and concerns is to look at what guidance is in place concerning CDT Code use:

- A third-party payer is supposed to use the code number (e.g., D0120), its nomenclature and its descriptor as written.
- The ADA defines procedure code bundling as "the systematic combining of distinct dental procedures by third-party payers that results in a reduced benefit for the patient/beneficiary." Procedure code bundling is frowned upon by the ADA.

  However, dentists who have signed participating provider agreements with third-party payers may be bound to plan provisions that limit or exclude coverage for concurrent procedures.
- The Health Insurance Portability and Accountability Act (HIPAA) requires the procedure code reported on a claim be from the CDT Code version that is effective on the date of service. Yet neither HIPAA, ADA policy nor the CDT Code itself require that a third-party payer cover every listed dental procedure.
- Covered dental procedures are identified in the contract between the plan purchaser and the third-party payer.

Many patients do not understand how dental benefit programs work and that coverage limitations and exclusions may limit reimbursement for necessary care. Such a misunderstanding is compounded when EOB language suggests that the dentist is at fault. Ensuring patients understand the limitations of their dental plan prior to treatment may help avoid problems and maintain a strong dentist-patient relationship.

Some dental claim adjudication practices are appropriate when based on plan design and should be clearly explained on the EOB to prevent misunderstandings. Other situations, where the EOB message suggests the dentist is in error, may pose problems. Each of these conditions is illustrated in the following examples:

- **Acceptable EOB explanation**: A claim for a "D4355 full mouth debridement" and a two-surface restoration is adjudicated, and only the D4355 is reimbursed. The EOB message states that the benefit plan has limitations and exclusions, one of which is that the plan does not cover any restorative procedure delivered on the same day as a D4355. In this example, the payer has not paid for the procedure due to benefit plan design limitations – there is no suggestion that the dentist has done anything improper.

- **Unacceptable EOB explanation**: The dentist reports a D1110 on the claim because the patient is 13 years old with predominantly adult dentition, but the EOB lists D1120 with a message that this is the correct code for a patient under the age of 15. In this example, the payer is wrong, as the message implies that the dentist reported the incorrect prophylaxis procedure code. Here the payer ignored the CDT Code's descriptor where dentition, not age, is the criterion for reporting an adult versus child prophylaxis. What the payer should do when the benefit plan specifies an age-based benefit limitation is accept the claim as submitted and note on the EOB that the claim has been adjudicated based on benefit plan design.

The second example illustrates why it is important that the dental office help the patient understand the clinical basis for treatment. In this case, the type of prophylaxis is determined by the state of the patient's dentition, not age, even though the patient's benefit may be determined by age.

Dental benefit plan limitations and exclusions affect how a claim is adjudicated and, as noted above, a payer may reject or not reimburse a claim in accordance with the benefit plan's provisions. Just as benefit plan designs vary, there is variation in participating provider contract provisions, and if you have one (or more) each must be reviewed to see how claim submission and processing may be affected. The ADA Contract Analysis Service, an ADA member benefit, can identify areas of provider contract provisions that may be of concern and be addressed before signing the contract. More information on the Contract Analysis Service is available here: ***ADA.org/en/member-center/member-benefits/legal-resources/contract-analysis-service***.

Participating provider contracts are between the dentist and payer. These contracts may include provisions that require you to accept least expensive alternative treatment (LEAT) reimbursement, or agree to reimbursement based on payer guidelines instead of specific procedure codes reported on a claim. A dentist who signs a participating provider contract is generally bound to its legally sound provisions. Likewise, the payer is also bound to the contract provisions and cannot obligate you to do something that is beyond the signed agreement.

It is appropriate to appeal the benefit decision if you think the claim has not been properly adjudicated. When appealing a claim, it is important to follow the specific instructions provided by the particular carrier including the submittal of the appeal in writing within the time allowed by the carrier. It is important to send it to the specified department of the carrier and it must be in the required format. The word "appeal" should prominently appear in the title and text of the document, as well as in any cover letter that accompanies the appeal document.

Remember, the dentist consultant representing the carrier may only be looking at a dental claim form and you will want to provide the consultant as much information as possible so that he or she will agree with your treatment plan and approve the appropriate benefits for your patient.

A proper appeal involves sending the carrier a written request to reconsider the claim. Additional documentation should be included to give the carrier a clearer picture of why you recommended the treatment. For example, the following claim attachments may assist in getting consideration for core buildup claims – radiographic evidence of the need for a buildup, and a narrative description providing as much explanatory information as possible (even if this appears obvious to you). If you have further questions, it is best to give that carrier a call.

Remember, you are trying to have the dentist consultant understand the rationale for your recommended treatment plan so that your patient can receive the appropriate benefit from his or her plan.

It may help to ask the dentist consultant to call you if the claim is going to be denied. This way you can discuss the case with the dentist consultant on a professional level. You may want to leave a time and date when you will be available so that the consultant does not call while you are seeing patients.

Payers using the CDT Code must be licensed to do so – and abide by the copyright license. Any payer actions that do not adhere to contractual obligations may represent misuse, and be reason to seek redress. The copyright license does not dictate how a procedure code is to be reimbursed and cannot be used as a tool to force payers to use the CDT Code in a particular manner.

However, arbitrary payer action is an ongoing ADA concern and we ask that dentists report such actions so that staff can address recurring issues with the third-party payer involved. Also, it is appropriate to appeal the benefit decision if you think the claim has not been properly adjudicated, and ADA staff is prepared to assist in your understanding of the appeal process.

Even if an objectionable use of the CDT Code is not a license violation or illegal, ADA staff remains available to contact third-party payers, attempting to discuss the issues and to resolve potential conflicts. Dentist reports of concerns enable ADA staff to address individual issues with payers, as well as providing the means to determine, monitor and address patterns of payer actions.

Note: The ADA Member Service Center (MSC) is your first point of contact when you have questions about the CDT Code and its use, or to report possible third-party payer "misuse." Please contact the MSC by telephone at 312.440.2500.

If you wish to simply alert the ADA to a concern, you can complete the downloadable form on *ADA.org* titled, "third-party payer complaint form" which gives dental offices the opportunity to provide information on the problems experienced with third-party payers.

This form was developed by the ADA Center for Dental Benefits, Coding and Quality to track industry trends and facilitate discussions with dental benefit plans and benefits administrators. The form is available online at:

success.ada.org/en/dental-benefits/online-third-party-form

The "Golden Rules" of Procedure Coding

Correct coding, part and parcel of the following rules, demonstrates a dentist's adherence to the ADA's Principles of Ethics and Code of Professional Conduct, particularly "5.A. Representation of Care" that states "Dentists shall not represent the care being rendered to their patients in a false or misleading manner."

- "Code for what you do" is the fundamental rule to apply in all coding situations.
- After reading the full nomenclature and descriptor, select the code that matches the procedure delivered to the patient.
- If there is no applicable code, document the service using an unspecified, by report ("999") code, and include a clear and appropriate narrative.
- The existence of a procedure code does not mean that the procedure is a covered or reimbursed benefit in a dental benefit plan.
- Treatment planning is based on clinical need, not covered services.

If you have difficulty finding an appropriate CDT code consider whether there may be another way to describe the procedure. The CDT Manual's alphabetic index, and the glossary of dental terms posted on *ADA.org* are likely to be helpful in these situations.

Code Changes in CDT 2019

The number and nature of annual CDT Code changes vary, as does their relevance to an individual dentist vary – primarily based on her or his type of practice. CDT 2019 incorporates a variety of CDT Code entry actions – 15 additions, five revisions, four deletions, and 2 editorial – summarized in the following table.

Code	Addition **Revision, Deletion,** Editorial
I. Diagnostic	
D0412	Addition
II. Preventive	
~~D1515~~	Deletion
D1516	Addition
D1517	Addition
~~D1525~~	Deletion
D1526	Addition
D1527	Addition
III. Restorative	
None	
IV. Endodontics	
None	
V. Periodontics	
D4230	Editorial
D4231	Editorial
VI. Prosthodontics (removable)	
D5211	**Revision**
D5212	**Revision**
~~D5281~~	Deletion
D5282	Addition
D5283	Addition
D5630	**Revision**
D5876	Addition
VII. Maxillofacial Prosthetics	
None	
VIII. Implant Services	
None	
IX. Prosthodontics, fixed	
None	
X. Oral and Maxillofacial Surgery	
D7283	**Revision**
XI. Orthodontics	
None	

Code	Addition Revision, Deletion, Editorial
XI. Adjunctive General Services	
D9130	Addition
D9219	**Revision**
D9613	Addition
~~D9940~~	Deletion
D9944	Addition
D9945	Addition
D9946	Addition
D9961	Addition
D9990	Addition

Some of the CDT 2019 changes listed in this table are stand alone and others – additions with associated revisions or deletions – are interrelated. These changes will be addressed in detail within the following chapters.

Substantive Changes: What and Why

There are substantive changes that reflect how the CDT Code evolves to accommodate procedure documentation needs by adding new or revising existing code entries. The three most notable of these and rationales for their inclusion in CDT 2019 follow in category of service order. All are color coded in blue.

D0100-D0999 Diagnostic

New entry:

D0412 blood glucose level test – in-office using a glucose meter

Rationale for the addition from submitter's action request form:

As diabetes is one of the most common chronic diseases, practicing dentists are likely to encounter it frequently. If a diabetic dental patient is about to undergo a long complex procedure, it is essential to know what their blood sugar level is at that moment. Even though the patient's A1C percentage may be at an acceptable control level, the patient's actual blood sugar level at that moment may actually be very low, and heading toward a hypoglycemic event.

By checking their current blood sugar level with a glucometer (which cannot be obtained via an A1C test), prior to a complex procedure, it might be realized that the patient's blood sugar level is below 70mg/dl, and the procedure should not be initiated at that time, as a hypoglycemic event is likely to occur during the procedure, putting the patient at great risk. On the other hand, the patient's current blood sugar level may be over 300 mg/dl, even though their A1C level is at an acceptable percentage. Any elective surgical procedures should be avoided at that time, as such a high level of blood glucose could lead to delayed healing of the surgical site and severe infection.

Glucometer testing would also be utilized for individuals who have risk factors for diabetes, but who have not been diagnosed with either pre-diabetes or diabetes. Moreover, staff should be trained to recognize the signs of hypoglycemia and treat patients who become hypoglycemic.

D9000-D9999 Adjunctive General Services

New entry:

D9613 infiltration of sustained release therapeutic drug – single or multiple sites
Infiltration of a sustained release pharmacologic agent for long acting surgical site pain control. Not for local anesthesia purposes.

Rationale for the addition from submitter's action request form:

With the increased focus on the use of opioids and the problems associated with their use patients are requesting non-narcotic alternatives for post-operative pain control. Doctors are now utilizing a sustained release pharmacologic agent infiltrated at the surgical site to reduce the use of narcotic pain medicine in their pain management protocol.

The use of an injectable non-opioid therapeutic sustained release drug around the surgical site at the end of a procedure has been shown to be effective in reducing or eliminating the need for post-operative opioids for pain control.

D9990 certified translation or sign language services – per visit

Rationale for the addition from submitter's action request form:

With the implementation in 2016 of the Affordable Care Act, Section 1557 regarding non-discrimination, there is a requirement for covered entities to provide free language services to people whose primary language is not English. We believe translation services warrants its own code to improve efficiencies in benefit determination.

Currently translation services is only part of a long list of services within code D9994, and there is no means for an office to indicate that this service was provided without a request for additional information. Having a dedicated code improves processing efficiencies and enables benefit determinations be made without additional documentation. This will provide greater efficiency for both providers and third-party payers.

There are 21 other substantive changes in CDT 2019. Each will be fully addressed in its applicable CDT 2019 Companion category chapter:

Chapter	Substantive Change	
Preventive	~~**D1515**~~	~~**space maintainer – fixed - bilateral**~~
	<u>**D1516**</u>	<u>**space maintainer – fixed – bilateral, maxillary**</u>
	<u>**D1517**</u>	<u>**space maintainer – fixed – bilateral, mandibular**</u>
	~~**D1525**~~	~~**space maintainer – removable – bilateral**~~
	<u>**D1526**</u>	<u>**space maintainer – removable – bilateral, maxillary**</u>
	<u>**D1527**</u>	<u>**space maintainer – removable – bilateral, mandibular**</u>
Prosthodontics, fixed	**D5211**	**maxillary partial denture – resin base (including** ~~**any conventional clasps**~~ <u>**retentive/clasping materials,**</u> **rests, and teeth)** ~~Includes acrylic resin base denture with resin or wrought wire clasps.~~
	D5212	**mandibular partial denture – resin base (including** ~~**any conventional clasps**~~ <u>**retentive/clasping materials,**</u> **rests, and teeth)** ~~Includes acrylic resin base denture with resin or wrought wire clasps.~~
	~~**D5281**~~	~~**removable unilateral partial denture – one piece cast metal (including clasps and teeth)**~~
	<u>**D5282**</u>	<u>**removable unilateral partial denture – one piece cast metal (including clasps and teeth), maxillary**</u>
	<u>**D5283**</u>	<u>**removable unilateral partial denture – one piece cast metal (including clasps and teeth), mandibular**</u>
	D5630	**repair or replace broken** ~~**clasp**~~ <u>**retentive/clasping materials**</u> **per tooth**
	<u>**D5876**</u>	<u>**add metal substructure to acrylic full denture (per arch)**</u>

Chapter	Substantive Change
Oral and Maxillofacial Surgery	**D7283 placement of device to facilitate eruption of impacted tooth** Placement of an ~~orthodontic bracket, band or other device~~ attachment on an unerupted tooth, after its exposure, to aid in its eruption. Report the surgical exposure separately using D7280.
Adjunctive General Services	**D9130 temporomandibular joint dysfunction – non-invasive physical therapies** Therapy including but not limited to massage, diathermy, ultrasound, or cold application to provide relief from muscle spasms, inflammation or pain, intending to improve freedom of motion and joint function. This should be reported on a per session basis. **D9219 evaluation for moderate sedation, deep sedation or general anesthesia** ~~**D9940 occlusal guard, by report**~~ ~~Removable dental appliances, which are designed to minimize the effects of bruxism (grinding) and other occlusal factors.~~ **D9944 occlusal guard – hard appliance, full arch** Removable dental appliance designed to minimize the effects of bruxism or other occlusal factors. Not to be reported for any type of sleep apnea, snoring or TMD appliances. **D9945 occlusal guard – soft appliance, full arch** Removable dental appliance designed to minimize the effects of bruxism or other occlusal factors. Not to be reported for any type of sleep apnea, snoring or TMD appliances. **D9946 occlusal guard – hard appliance, partial arch** Removable dental appliance designed to minimize the effects of bruxism or other occlusal factors. Provides only partial occlusal coverage such as anterior deprogrammer. Not to be reported for any type of sleep apnea, snoring or TMD appliances. **D9961 duplicate/copy patient's records**

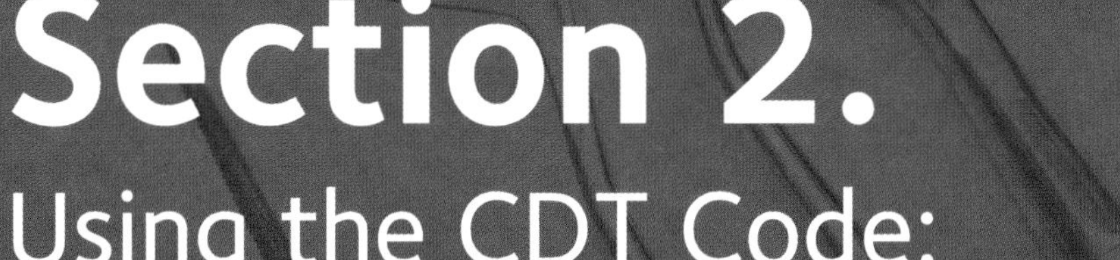

Section 2.

Using the CDT Code: Definitions and Key Concepts, Coding Scenarios and Coding Q&A

Section 2
Using the CDT Code: Definitions and Key Concepts, Coding Scenarios and Coding Q&A

Introduction

Individual chapters in this section, including one for each of the CDT Code's 12 categories of service, contain definitions of key terms, information on notable changes, clinical scenarios, and Q&A based on real-life situations. Answers to these questions and scenarios illustrate coding solutions for the situations described. These scenarios and solutions reflect common and accepted practices, but may not reflect the way your office would manage a given situation. The dentist who treats a patient is the person who can best determine appropriate treatment and the CDT codes that best describe it.

The scenarios and Q&A are the product of questions received from ADA members and developed by ADA staff, as well as based on the contributions of chapter authors. They are not to be considered legal advice or a guarantee that individual payer contracts will follow this assistance.

Use this information to get a better understanding of the principles of reporting using the CDT Code. Since it covers subjects from many different perspectives, it is likely that some will be more applicable to your particular situation than others. All the scenarios and Q&A, including those that involve procedures you may not usually report, are of value since the principles demonstrated can often be applied to areas of your practice.

Chapter 1.
D0100 – D0999 Diagnostic

By Ralph A. Cooley, D.D.S.

Introduction

Dentists and other dental health care providers dedicate years of their lives learning how to provide excellent oral health care to their patients. But just providing this quality of care is not enough. In today's world, one must have a complete and accurate record of the care that is delivered. That is why the *Code on Dental Procedures and Nomenclature* (CDT Code) was established. In this chapter we will discuss key concepts and code changes, some common coding scenarios, and frequently asked questions about coding for diagnostic procedures.

Key Definitions and Concepts

Evaluation: The systematic determination or judgment about a condition, disease, or treatment.

Clinical oral evaluations: As with all ADA procedure codes, there is no distinction made between the evaluations provided by general practitioners and specialists. Report additional diagnostic and/or definitive procedures separately.

Imaging: Creating a visual representation of the interior of a body revealing inner structures that may have been blocked by skin or bone.

Intraoral image: A visual representation of the mouth derived by placing a film, plate, or sensor within the mouth.

Extraoral image: A visual representation of the mouth derived by placing a film, plate, or sensor outside the mouth.

Changes to This Category

One code was added in CDT 2019's Diagnostic category:

D0412 blood glucose level test – in-office using a glucose meter
This procedure provides an immediate finding of a patient's blood glucose level at the time of sample collection for the point-of-service analysis.

There were no revisions, deletions, or editorial changes.

Diagnosis Codes – ICD-10-CM

The CDT to ICD tables in Appendix 1 provide appropriate guidance on linkages between Diagnostic procedure codes and diagnosis codes.

Please note that the International Classification of Disease (ICD) is a code set where letters and numbers are given to every diagnosis, description of symptoms and causes of death attributed to the human species, and ICD-10-CM became effective on October 1, 2015. Dentists should know that ICD coding is becoming more accepted by state Medicaid programs with some states requiring the use of an ICD code for the diagnosis along with a CDT code when dental treatment is rendered. The current ADA Dental Claim Form and the HIPAA standard electronic dental claim transaction can report up to four diagnosis codes.

CODING SCENARIO #1

Patient Age 11 – Evaluation, Preventive, and Orthodontic Services

A new patient, age 11, was seen for a first exam, cleaning, and fluoride varnish application. During the exam, the dentist noted that the erupting tooth #4 was impinging on the band loop spacer that another dentist cemented to #3 and decided to remove it.

How might this visit be coded?

D0150 comprehensive oral evaluation – new or established patient

D1120 prophylaxis – child

D1206 topical application of fluoride varnish

D1555 removal of fixed space maintainer

Note: If in this scenario, if the topical fluoride was a rinse or other appropriate in-office fluoride application other than a varnish, **D1206** would not be correct. The appropriate CDT code would be:

D1208 topical application of fluoride – excluding varnish

But what if the same patient was not new and the doctor had placed the space maintainer two years ago? How would this encounter be coded?

D0120 periodic oral evaluation

D1120 prophylaxis – child

D1206 topical application of fluoride varnish

The exam, in this case, would be periodic (**D0120**) because the patient was seen previously, but the prophylaxis and fluoride codes remain the same. **D1555** is not used to report space maintainer removal in this alternative scenario as the code's descriptor specifies that it is for a dentist who did not place the space maintainer.

CODING SCENARIO #2

New Patient with Diagnostic Gathering Challenges and Tobacco Use

A 21-year-old new patient is seen for a first exam. You note that he has numerous decayed anterior and posterior teeth but when you attempt to take a full mouth intraoral series of radiographs you discover he has a severe gag response. You take a panoramic image and 2 extra oral bitewings.

He is also a heavy chewing tobacco user so you perform a tissue fluorescence oral cancer exam and spend about 15 minutes discussing his tobacco use, what it is doing to his mouth, and his options to try to quit.

How would you code this visit?

D0150 comprehensive oral evaluation

D0330 panoramic radiographic image

D0251 extra-oral posterior radiographic image

Choosing the panoramic (D0330) and extra-oral bitewing (D0251) radiographs allowed you to get a preliminary understanding of his oral conditions. Note: this is not a "full mouth series" because these are not intraoral radiographic images. The dentist may consider utilizing some alternative methods to aid in capturing some intraoral images later.

Codes for the tissue fluorescence oral cancer exam and counseling the patient for his tobacco use are:

D0431 adjunctive pre-diagnostic test that aids in detection of mucosal abnormalities including premalignant and malignant lesions, not to include cytology or biopsy procedures

Note: Examples of adjunctive pre-diagnostic tests that aid in detection of mucosal abnormalities may include VELscope, OralID, MicorLux DL, or VizLite Plus. This test is done in addition to your normal visual and palpation exam that is part of a comprehensive evaluation.

D1320 tobacco counseling for the control and prevention of oral disease

CODING SCENARIO #3

Child Under Three – Evaluation and Parent Counseling, and Preventive Services

Note: The American Academy of Pediatric Dentistry and the ADA advise that children should have their first dental visit within six months of the eruption of the first primary tooth.

The doctor performed an intraoral examination on a one-year-old patient while the mother restrained the child's forehead in her lap. The dentist determined that the child had maxillary and mandibular primary incisors and that they were caries free. The dentist also removed plaque using an ultra-soft toothbrush and applied fluoride varnish. The doctor explained to the parent how to use a washcloth or soft brush to remove plaque each day and the importance of getting the child to go to sleep without a bottle. They discussed foods that can "lead to decay" (caries) and recommended that she return in a year for an exam after most of the primary teeth have erupted.

Here is what occurred during the child's first dental visit:

- Oral examination
- Toothbrush deplaquing
- Fluoride varnish
- Discussion of diet and preventive care with the parent

How would you code this first visit?

D0145 oral evaluation for a patient under three years of age and counseling with primary caregiver

D1120 prophylaxis – child

D1206 topical application of fluoride varnish

Note: The evaluation and counseling code (**D0145**):

- has both diagnostic and preventive characteristics
- is specifically for children under three years of age
- includes an evaluation of oral conditions, history, and caries susceptibility
- includes development of an oral hygiene regimen
- always includes counseling the primary caregiver or parent

What evaluation code could be used on the next visit?

Either the same evaluation and counseling code (**D0145**) or the periodic evaluation code (**D0120**) could be used for the next visit. There is nothing in the **D0145** nomenclature or descriptor that precludes its use for more than one visit, as long as the patient is still under three years of age and all the components of the procedure are completed. The periodic exam might be appropriate as the primary dentition develops and if the other criteria are not met. The prophylaxis and fluoride would remain the same.

CODING SCENARIO #4

Radiographs – What Constitutes a Full Mouth Series?

The descriptor to procedure code **D0210** defines a complete series of radiographic images, as seen in the CDT manual's entry:

D0210 intraoral – complete series of radiographic images
A radiographic survey of the whole mouth, usually consisting of 14-22 periapical and posterior bitewing images intended to display the crowns and roots of all teeth, periapical areas and alveolar bone.

Note: The descriptor was drawn from The Selection of Patients for X-Ray Examinations: Dental Radiographic Examinations published by the FDA in 2004.

With this in mind, consider how radiographs for patients A, B, C, and D are documented.

Patient A is missing all second and third molars

The office takes ten periapical x-rays: three upper anterior, three lower anterior and one posterior in each quadrant.

If the radiographs display the crowns and roots of all teeth, periapical areas and alveolar bone crest, the full mouth series procedure code **D0210** would be appropriate, even though Patient A's radiographs do not include bitewing. According to the descriptor bitewings are included when indicated, but they are not a required component of this procedure.

If the radiographs do not display the crowns and roots of all teeth, periapical areas and alveolar bone crest, the applicable procedure codes are:

D0220 intraoral – periapical first radiographic image (reported once)

D0230 intraoral – periapical each additional radiographic image (reported nine times)

Patient B has all her teeth and has impacted partially erupted third molars

The office takes a panoramic x-ray and four posterior bitewings.

D0330 panoramic radiographic image

D0274 bitewings – four radiographic images

Since a panoramic radiographic image is not intraoral, this combination could not correctly be reported as a full mouth series (**D0210**).

Note: The ADA Council on Dental Benefit Programs receives many calls stating that claims for **D0330** and **D0274** are downcoded by third-party payers to **D0210** for purposes of reimbursement. This term *downcoding* is defined in the Glossary published on *ADA.org* as:

> **downcoding**: A practice of third-party payers in which the benefit code has been changed to a less complex and/or lower cost procedure than was reported, except where delineated in contract agreements.

Patient C has a maxillary full denture and fourteen mandibular teeth

The office takes four periapicals of the upper edentulous ridge, seven periapicals of the lower arch and four posterior bitewings. This situation, while not the most common scenario, does meet all the criteria for and is correctly coded as a full mouth series.

D0210 intraoral – complete series of radiographic images
A radiographic survey of the whole mouth, usually consisting of 14-22 periapical and posterior bitewing images intended to display the crowns and roots of all teeth, periapical areas and alveolar bone.

Patient D is edentulous in the mandible, and has six remaining teeth in the maxillary arch: teeth # 6, 7, 8, 9, 10, and 11

A panoramic film and four periapicals were taken in the maxillary anterior region.

This situation would not be coded as a D0210 complete series because there was not an intraoral radiographic image of the whole mouth. It would be coded as:

D0330 panoramic radiographic image

D0220 intraoral – periapical first radiographic image (reported once)

D0230 intraoral – periapical each additional radiographic image (reported three times)

Regardless of the patient's dental benefit plan, the reporting of performed procedures should always reflect what treatment was provided. Alternate payment provisions may apply, but the third-party should send statements to patients and providers alike to explain why an alternate benefit was provided.

Dentists who have signed provider agreements with third-party payers should check their contracts to see if there are provisions that apply to this situation.

CODING SCENARIO #5

Oral Cancer – An Enhanced Examination

An oral cancer evaluation is included in the descriptors of both of the comprehensive oral evaluations (**D0150** and **D0180**) and the periodic oral evaluation (**D0120**). Visual inspection using operatory lighting and palpation are the techniques that are frequently used in routine oral cancer evaluations. A dentist may decide that patients with increased cancer risk factors should also receive an enhanced oral cancer examination, one that is more extensive than a routine oral cancer screening and may include the use of additional diagnostic aids.

How could the dentist report use of additional diagnostic aids in the oral cancer examination?

There is not an independent code for an enhanced oral cancer examination, but there is a code that can be used when some type of staining or similar procedure is performed:

D0431 adjunctive pre-diagnostic test that aids in detection of mucosal abnormalities including premalignant and malignant lesions, not to include cytology or biopsy procedures

This code may be used to report the use of the following:

- Tissue reflectance (e.g., Vizilite Plus®, MicorLux DL)
- Autofluorescence (e.g. VELscope, OralID)
- Any intraoral vital staining technique (e.g., toluidine blue)

If the additional procedures are not described by **D0431** the dentist could use:

D0999 unspecified diagnostic procedure, by report

D0999 can be used to report any diagnostic procedure which does not seem to be included in the CDT Code. A narrative that describes the service must be included on the claim when this code is used.

CODING SCENARIO #6

Orthognathic Surgery Planning

An oral and maxillofacial surgery office recently installed a cone beam radiography machine. It was used to treatment plan some anticipated orthognathic surgery for a patient. Following image capture, several axial and lateral views were consulted to plan the surgery. A panoramic view was also produced to send to the patient's orthodontist.

After consultation with the orthodontist, the surgeon constructed a 3D virtual model, which they viewed together on the computer, to properly locate a temporary implant to anchor the orthodontic appliance. The virtual model could be manipulated on the screen to allow them to visualize other anatomical structures in the area and their relationship to the teeth to determine the ideal location to place the implant.

A transmucosal endosseous implant was placed as a temporary fixation device for the patient's braces. The temporary implant will be removed when orthodontic treatment is completed.

How could you code the initial treatment planning visit's diagnostic imaging procedures?

D0367 cone beam CT capture and interpretation with field of view of both jaws; with or without cranium

This code was added effective January 1, 2013 specifically to report procedures related to cone beam imaging technology. It replaced the separate cone beam data capture (**D0360**) and two-dimension reconstruction (**D0362**) codes. The image capture includes two-dimensional sectional (tomographic) views from the axial (coronal or frontal) and lateral (sagittal) planes, as well as the panoramic view.

How could you code the subsequent consultation? (3D virtual model)

D0393 treatment simulation using 3D image volume

The 3D virtual model is a three-dimensional image reconstructed from data acquired during the treatment planning visit.

CODING SCENARIO #7

Temporomandibular Joint (TMJ) Disorder Treatment

A patient, referred to the dental office by her ear, nose and throat (ENT) physician, has a history of constant headaches and facial pain. The ENT saw no sinus related issues after a thorough examination including radiographic images. After completing a comprehensive oral evaluation (**D0150**), the dentist recognized the patient's symptoms as a temporomandibular disorder of significant complexity. The patient exhibited limited opening and was in discomfort every morning.

Further evaluation was needed to diagnose this condition and that examination included listening to the joint with a stethoscope, detailed palpation of all the muscles of mastication, recording of occlusal relationships, ranges of motion, and areas of musculoskeletal tenderness.

The dentist did an extensive review of the patient's lifestyle, including stress coping mechanisms. She identified many potential contributing factors to the TMD condition. Teeth #18 and #19 were missing and tooth #15 had super-erupted to the point where the patient could not close without moving his jaw to the right. A tongue thrust habit resulted in a severe anterior open bite, and there was extensive incisal wear on all anterior teeth.

The doctor decided that following extraction of #15, an orthotic TMJ appliance covering the mandibular occlusal surfaces would allow the patient to reposition his jaw to a more comfortable position. It would also protect those teeth from increasing wear due to oral habits. After the patient was more comfortable, the doctor believed that a comprehensive treatment plan could be made.

How would the recent diagnostic visit be coded?

Due to the limited scope, the doctor can choose one of two problem-focused evaluations:

D0140 limited oral evaluation – problem focused

or **D0160 detailed and extensive oral evaluation – problem focused, by report**

In this case, the nature and complexity of the problems suggest that **D0160** would be the most appropriate code for this evaluation. Use of this code requires submission of a narrative report.

CODING SCENARIO #8

Treating a Patient Suffering From Swelling, Pain and Periodontal Disease

A patient presented in pain and complaining about swelling around one particular tooth. The doctor's emergency evaluation focused on the patient's complaint and included two periapical radiographic images and pocket measurements of the teeth in the area. The swelling was clearly adjacent to tooth #3 and there was bleeding and exudate upon probing.

The doctor treated the patient for a periodontal abscess by gross debridement and draining through the sulcus, irrigating the pocket with chlorhexidine and prescribing the patient an antibiotic.

How could this encounter be coded?

Since the evaluation was both problem-focused and limited to the patient's complaint, the appropriate codes for diagnostic procedures would be:

D0140 limited oral evaluation – problem focused

D0220 intraoral – periapical first radiographic image

D0230 intraoral – periapical each additional radiographic image

In this case there are several codes that might be used to document the operative services, alone or in combination. Three possible procedure coding options are:

D9110 palliative (emergency) treatment of dental pain – minor procedure
This is typically reported on a "per visit" basis for emergency treatment of dental pain.

Note: **D9110** is a "catch-all" code that covers a broad array of procedures.

D7510 incision and drainage of abscess – intraoral soft tissue
Involves incision through mucosa, including periodontal origins.

Note: Discussions at the Code Maintenance Committee (CMC) meetings indicated that **D7510** was considered to be appropriate even when "incision" is made through the gingival sulcus.

D4342 periodontal scaling and root planing – one to three teeth, per quadrant

Note: The descriptor for **D4342** indicates that it is a "definitive procedure." Therefore, it may not be the appropriate code when the procedure is only managing acute conditions.

CODING SCENARIO #9

A Partially Edentulous Patient with Bleeding Gums, Rampant Calculus, and White Lesions

Patient presented with massive accretion of calculus on teeth also covered by a dark brown veneer of coffee and tobacco residue. The calculus effectively cemented a lower partial in place that the doctor wished to remove. An ultrasonic scaler was the doctor's instrument of choice for calculus removal before a comprehensive oral evaluation, which would be delivered during a subsequent appointment.

After the full mouth debridement was completed there were additional diagnostic procedures: radiographs of the entire lower arch including four posterior and two anterior periapicals; two bitewings on the left and one on the right side; and a panoramic radiographic image.

Today's treatment included:

- initial evaluation that establishes the need for the gross removal of plaque and calculus
- gross removal of calculus and stain
- radiographs (6 PA, 3 BW, and 1 Panoramic)
- disaggregated transepithelial biopsy (brush) of white patch
- dispensing one 16 oz. bottle of chlorhexidine gluconate rinse

How would the five services delivered during today's encounter be coded?

Initial evaluation:

D0191 assessment of a patient
A limited clinical inspection that is performed to identify possible signs of oral or systemic disease, malformation, or injury, and the potential need for referral for diagnosis and treatment.

or **D0140 limited oral evaluation – problem focused**
An evaluation limited to a specific oral health problem or complaint. This may require interpretation of information acquired through additional diagnostic procedures. Report additional diagnostic procedures separately. Definitive procedures may be required on the same date as the evaluation.

Typically, patients receiving this type of evaluation present with a specific problem or dental emergencies, trauma, acute infections, etc.

Gross removal of calculus and stain:

D4355 full mouth debridement to enable a comprehensive oral evaluation and diagnosis on a subsequent visit
Full mouth debridement involves the preliminary removal of plaque and calculus that interferes with the ability of the dentist to perform a comprehensive oral evaluation. Not to be completed on the same day as D0150, D0160, or D0180.

Note: This procedure is done prior to completing diagnosis when it is not possible to adequately access tooth surfaces and periodontal areas because of excessive plaque and calculus.

Radiographs (6 PA, 3 BW, and Panoramic):

These nine radiographs and the panoramic radiographic image do not match the CDT Code's definition of a "full mouth series" added as the "D0210 intraoral — complete series" procedure code effective January 1, 2009. Therefore, the radiographs in this scenario would be reported using the panoramic, periapical and bitewing codes:

D0220 intraoral — periapical first radiographic image

D0230 intraoral — periapical each additional radiographic image

Note: Report D0230 five times, once for each additional radiographic image.

D0273 bitewings — three radiographic images

D0330 panoramic radiographic image

Disaggregated transepithelial biopsy of white patch:

D7288 brush biopsy — transepithelial sample collection

Note: The brush biopsy samples disaggregated dermal and epithelial cells. A positive sample usually requires follow-up with an architecturally intact incisional or excisional sample.

Dispense one 16 oz. bottle of chlorhexidine gluconate rinse:

D9630 drugs or medicaments dispensed in the office for home use

Note: This code was revised in CDT 2017 to clarify that the procedure is dispensing in the office, and eliminates the requirement for a narrative report.

CODING SCENARIO #10

Preventive Resin Restorations

The patient arrived at the office for a recall visit. On the previous recall visit six months ago, this patient had nutritional counseling as well as several teeth that needed to be restored due to decay.

Before doing anything the doctor decided that a caries risk assessment should be completed, using the form posted on *ADA.org*. A look at the answers on the form – especially the combination of frequent consumption of soft drinks and energy drinks, past interproximal restorations, and two incipient carious lesions – led to the conclusion that the patient is at high risk of continuing caries development.

What is the appropriate CDT code to document the caries risk procedure?

D0603 caries risk assessment and documentation, with a finding of high risk
Using recognized assessment tools.

Note: Caries risk assessment information, including the updated tools, is available online at *ADA.org/en/member-center/oral-health-topics/caries-risk-assessment-and-management*. When a patient receives a caries risk assessment, the procedure is documented and reported with the CDT code whose nomenclature includes the identified level of risk:

D0601 caries risk assessment and documentation, with a finding of low risk

D0602 caries risk assessment and documentation, with a finding of moderate risk

D0603 caries risk assessment and documentation, with a finding of high risk

During the oral exam the doctor did indeed see what appeared to be small, carious, cavitated lesions on the occlusal surfaces of teeth # 30 and 31. After opening the lesions using a handpiece and removing caries, both preparations were very slight, ending in enamel, and did not extend into the dentin.

The doctor concluded that a minimally invasive restorative technique would be appropriate for this situation. A composite resin would be used to restore tooth form and function along with an unfilled resin used afterwards to seal out all the radiating grooves.

What CDT code would be appropriate to document this minimally invasive procedure?

D1352 preventive resin restoration in a moderate to high caries risk patient – permanent tooth

Note: The doctor knows that **D2391** (one surface posterior composite) is not appropriate since the dentin was untouched. Likewise, **D1351** (sealant – per tooth) isn't applicable since decay was present.

D1352 was added to the Code on Dental Procedures and Nomenclature effective January 1, 2011. It was added to enable documentation of a conservative restorative procedure where caries, erosion or other conditions affect the natural form and function of the tooth. This procedure is part of many dental school curricula under names that vary by school and region (e.g., preventive resin restoration; conservative resin restoration; or minimally invasive resin restoration).

CODING SCENARIO #11

Reactivated Recall Patient

A 51-year-old patient finally returns to the dental office after a two-year hiatus. Previously this patient (with a full complement of teeth) had been seen on a six-month basis with generalized 2-3 mm recession, periodontal pocket depths of 2-4 mm, and a propensity to build up supra-gingival calculus quickly. After performing a full mouth exam, including periodontal readings, most posterior teeth probe at 4-5 mm with some localized 6 mm and nearly 100 percent of the areas exhibit bleeding upon probing.

A full mouth radiographic series was taken two years ago, and the decision is made to take four bitewings. The patient reports increased fatigue and notes that all the nicks and scrapes received from being a mechanic "don't seem to heal as quickly this past year." The patient has not seen their MD in over two years but was previously informed that they were a borderline diabetic with no treatment recommended. The rest of the medical history is unremarkable with no medications being taken, but the patient appears to weigh much more than when last seen.

On the last dental visit, an HbA1c test was performed and recorded at 7.4%. Today, the test is given again and reads 7.9%. Due to the elevation of the HbA1c and worsening periodontal condition, the patient is advised to see their physician and a consult form is sent as well. The patient sees the physician and schedules for two subsequent appointments for scaling and root planning for all four quadrants. A third visit is scheduled for periodontal re-evaluation four to six weeks after the last SRP appointment and another HbA1c test.

How would you code today's appointment along with any subsequent treatment and follow up appointment?

Visit #1

D0180 comprehensive periodontal evaluation- new or established patient

D0274 bitewings – four radiographic images

D0411 HbA1c in office point of testing

Visit #2 (SRP two quadrants)

D4341 periodontal scaling and root planning- four or more teeth per quadrant (report twice)

Visit #3 (SRP two quadrants)

D4341 periodontal scaling and root planning- four or more teeth per quadrant (report twice)

Visit #4 (four to six weeks after completion of SRP and about three months after the first visit)

D0171 re-evaluation-post operative office visit

D0411 HbA1c in office point of testing
(This code entry does not include any guidance on frequency of delivery; third-party payer reimbursement will be based on benefit plan design.)

1. **I see there is a new code for an immediate finding of a patient's blood glucose level in the dental office using a glucose meter. Does that mean that this is necessary for every diabetic patient at every visit in my office?**

   The new code for testing of the blood glucose level of a patient in the dental office was adopted by the Code Maintenance Committee with a January 1, 2019 effective date. This enables the dental health care provider to code for this procedure but does not make any reference on when it should be done, and does not imply that it is necessary in every visit. The decision on whether to do this is determined by the judgment of the treating health care provider for each individual circumstance.

2. **Is it possible to use D0150 (comprehensive oral evaluation) again within 90 days after the initial visit to our dental office?**

   Reading the full CDT Code entry for D0150 will help determine whether the code is appropriate for documenting and reporting the procedure delivered to a patient. The D0150 descriptor states, in part, that this procedure (comprehensive oral examination) is applicable "to new patients, established patients who have a significant change in health conditions or other unusual circumstances, by report, or established patients who have been absent from active treatment for three or more years."

   Reporting the D0150 procedure would be appropriate if the patient had "a significant change in health conditions or other unusual circumstances." In that case, a narrative would accompany the code submission. If that were not the case with the patient, other oral evaluation codes such as D0140 limited oral evaluation-problem focused or D0160 detailed and extensive oral evaluation-problem-focused, by report may be more appropriate.

3. **My new panoramic imaging device enables me to acquire a single image that has the same, or more, diagnostic information than I see on multiple bitewing images. I've always considered a bitewing as an intra-oral image since the film is placed in the patient's mouth. With my new imaging device, the receptor is outside the oral cavity. What CDT code should I use now?**

   The ADA's online Glossary of Dental Clinical and Administrative Terms defines a bitewing radiograph as an "Interproximal radiographic view of the coronal portion of the tooth/teeth. A form of dental radiograph that may be taken with the long axis of the image oriented either horizontally or vertically, that reveals approximately the coronal halves of the maxillary and mandibular teeth and portions of the interdental alveolar septa on the same image." This definition opened the door to several coding options, such as "D0270 bitewing — single radiographic image" or "D0250 extra-oral — 2D projection radiographic image."

However, the CDT Code entry that more accurately describes the procedure is:

D0251 extra-oral posterior dental radiographic image
Image limited to exposure of complete posterior teeth in both dental arches. This is a unique image that is not derived from another image.

4. **My patient needs several extra-oral images to help diagnose the problem, but I do not see any code for additional images. What do I do?**

When reporting multiple extra-oral images the applicable procedure code is D0250, as revised in CDT 2016, with the number of images acquired noted in the "Qty." (Quantity) field on the claim form.

D0250 extra-oral — 2D projection radiographic image created using a stationary radiation source, and detector

5. **Are bitewings and a panoramic radiographic image considered a full mouth series of radiographs?**

No, these images are different from the "D0210 intraoral, complete series" procedure. According to the FDA's "The Selection of Patients for Dental Radiographic Examinations," published in 2004, a full mouth series is defined as "a set of intraoral radiographs usually consisting of 14 to 22 periapical and posterior bitewing images intended to display the crowns and roots of all teeth, periapical areas and alveolar bone crest." Effective January 1, 2009 this definition was incorporated into the D0210 descriptor.

Further, a panoramic radiographic image cannot be considered a full mouth series as it is an extra-oral film and it does not reflect the FDA definition of a full mouth series. Different procedure codes are available to report a full mouth series of radiographs (D0210) and a panoramic radiograph (D0330). Please note that bitewings taken as part of a full mouth series are not reported separately.

6. **Our office has begun to use new technology that provides 3D or 2D images of a patient that are generated from a CT-like scan. How do we code this?**

   Several procedure codes (e.g., D0364-D0368) are available to document "cone beam CT" diagnostic images taken in the dentist's office. There are separate codes based on the field of view. For example, an initial scan that yields coronal, sagittal, and panoramic views would be documented with:

   D0367 cone beam CT capture and interpretation with field of view of both jaws; with or without cranium
   The entire "cone beam" nomenclature must be read to determine which describes the diagnostic image.

7. **I've used D0350 to document oral/facial photographic images, but now I'm able to create both two- and three-dimensional photographic images. How do I document what I do when my diagnosis and treatment planning makes use of one or both types of images?**

   Changes effective with the publication of CDT 2015 enable you to document both 2D and 3D photographic images. There is a code for obtaining a 3D image as the procedure differs from acquiring a 2D image. D0350's nomenclature was revised to clarify that this procedure is applicable only to acquisition of 2D photographic images. The full CDT Code entries are:

   D0350 2D oral/facial photographic image obtained intra-orally or extra-orally

   D0351 3D photographic image
   This procedure is for dental or maxillofacial diagnostic purposes. It's not applicable for a CAD-CAM procedure.

8. **I took a panoramic image and extra-oral bitewings on a patient. Why wouldn't I code this as D0250 and on the claim report quantity of two?**

   The CDT 2016 contained a new procedure code for extra-oral bitewings, D0251. The correct coding from the Diagnostic Imaging section would be:

   D0330 panoramic radiographic image

   D0251 extra-oral posterior dental radiographic image

   Note: Include the number of D0251 images in the claim form's "Qty." field.

9. **When is it appropriate to report a consultation versus an evaluation procedure?**

   Typically, a consultation (D9310) is reported when one dentist refers a patient to another dentist for an opinion or advice on a particular problem encountered by the patient.

10. **Should the dentist who sees a patient referred by another dentist for an evaluation of a specific problem report a problem focused evaluation code (D0140; D0160), or the consultation code (D9310)? Also, does it matter if the dentist initiates treatment for the patient on the same visit?**

    Both D0140 and D0160 are both problem focused evaluations and either may be reported if the consulting dentist believes one or the other appropriately describes the service provided. Please note that neither of these evaluation procedures' nomenclatures or descriptors contain language that prohibits the consulting dentist from initiating and reporting additional services. These services are reported separately by their own unique codes.

    Code D9310 may be used if the consulting dentist believes it better describes the service provided when a patient is referred by another dentist for evaluation of a specific problem. According to this CDT code's descriptor, the dentist who is consulted may initiate additional diagnostic or therapeutic services for the patient, which are also reported separately by their own unique codes.

11. **When is it appropriate to report oral evaluation codes D0150, D0180, D0120 and D0140?**

    These four commonly reported codes are from the CDT Code's series of clinical evaluation codes (D0120 through D0180). Each one is thoroughly explained by their respective nomenclature and descriptor. For example:

    - The initial evaluation for a new patient may be reported using "D0150 comprehensive oral evaluation — new or established patient" or by "D0180 comprehensive periodontal evaluation — new or established patient."
    - If this patient becomes a patient of record returning after the initial evaluation, the service would be reported using "D0120 periodic oral evaluation-established patient".

- An evaluation of a patient who presents with a specific problem or dental emergency may be reported using "D0140 limited oral evaluation — problem focused."

Again, it is important to read the descriptor to distinguish what type of clinical oral evaluation is being coded for each particular patient visit.

12. Can I submit a periodic evaluation (D0120) on the same day as a full mouth debridement to enable comprehensive periodontal evaluation and diagnosis (D4355)?

According to its descriptor, D4355 is "not to be completed on the same day as D0150, D0160, or D0180." There is nothing in the descriptors of the oral evaluation code D0120 or D4355 that preclude reporting both on the same day. However, according to the ADA's Guide to Reporting Full Mouth Debridement, codes for patient assessment (D0191) or limited oral evaluation (D0140) procedures are more appropriate.

This is because D0120 descriptor includes actions that are also in the D0150 and D0180 descriptors, two procedures that the D4355 entry says cannot be reported on the same day. Also, benefit plans may have limitations or exclusions about paying for both D4355 and D0120 procedures when delivered on the same day.

13. We recently had a patient come in for a periodic oral evaluation. The doctor found signs and symptoms of periodontal disease and performed a complete periodontal evaluation. May I report both the periodic and periodontal evaluations since these are two separate procedures?

The comprehensive periodontal procedure D0180 includes all the components of a periodic evaluation D0120, and adds additional requirements for periodontal charting and the evaluation of periodontal conditions. When a patient presents with signs or symptoms of periodontal disease, and all these components are performed, D0180 would be reported.

14. May I submit a limited oral evaluation (D0140) and another procedure on the same day?

There is no language in the descriptor of D0140 that precludes the reporting of other procedures on the same date of service. However, some benefit plans have limitations or exclusions about paying for certain combinations of codes performed on the same day.

15. If seven vertical bitewings and a panoramic image are taken to show the entire oral cavity, can it be coded as a full mouth series D0210?

No. By definition of the descriptor of D0210, seven vertical bitewings and a panoramic radiographic image would not constitute a full mouth series (FMS) because the panoramic image is extra-oral and the intra-oral bitewings do not capture all of the structures of the entire mouth. It would be coded as:

D0330 panoramic radiographic image

D0277 vertical bitewings 7-8 radiographic images

16. Which CDT code could be used to document a periodontal re-evaluation, such as for monitoring post-operative tissue healing?

The following CDT code, added in CDT 2015, fills a coding gap as until then the only option was a "999" code:

D0171 re-evaluation — post operative office visit

17. Is reporting the "comprehensive periodontal evaluation" (D0180) limited to periodontists?

D0180 is not limited to periodontists. All dental procedure codes are available to any practitioner providing service within the scope of her or his license.

18. I have read the descriptors of the evaluation codes, but am confused as to which code should be reported when a very young child is evaluated in the office. None of them seem to apply. What should be reported?

The procedure code for the evaluation of a child under age three and including counseling of the child's primary caregiver may be reported. This code is "D0145 oral evaluation for a patient under three years of age and counseling with primary caregiver."

19. Can code D0145 be reported every time the child comes into the office for an evaluation, or should we report a recall evaluation for subsequent visits?

A separate evaluation code was added because of the unique procedures that are necessary when evaluating a very young child. Depending on the nature of the evaluation, a periodic evaluation (D0120) or an oral evaluation for a patient under three years of age (D0145) would be appropriate choices to consider.

20. Must a caries risk assessment procedure be performed and submitted on a third-party claim that includes an oral evaluation code?

The CDT Code does not support any third-party payer requirement that a caries risk assessment procedure, D0601-D0603, must be submitted with an oral evaluation procedure (e.g., D0120, D0145 or D0150). Any such requirement comes from the payer's reimbursement policies, or benefit plan limitations and exclusions.

21. Is a caries susceptibility test (D0425) the same as a caries detectability test?

No, they are different procedures. A caries susceptibility test is a diagnostic test for determining a patient's propensity for caries. There is no procedure code for a caries detectability test, which aids in determining the presence of caries. "D0999 unspecified diagnostic procedure, by report" may be used to report a caries detectability test.

22. Can I submit a code for pulp vitality tests or is this considered to be included in all endodontic procedures?

Yes, you may submit this as a separate service (D0460) as it is a stand-alone code. It includes multiple teeth and contra lateral comparison(s), as indicated.

23. Are radiographic images taken during endodontic procedures considered to be part of the procedure as well, or can they be coded for individually?

Any image taken prior to the start of endodontic therapy can be coded individually, but all endodontic therapies include intra-operative radiographs as part of the treatment.

24. Are there rules or regulations regarding in office HbA1c testing?

Yes, some states may consider this testing "Outside the scope of the state's Dental Practice Act," which could make it unlawful to perform this test. Also, federal rules may limit the type or brand of device that may be used.

25. I use a laser caries detection device sometimes to help diagnose incipient decay. Is there a code for this?

The following code, added in CDT 2017, would be applicable as the laser is considered part of the armamentarium that could be used to deliver the procedure.

D0600 non-ionizing diagnostic procedure capable of quantifying, monitoring, and recording changes in structure of enamel, dentin, and cementum

26. A patient was seen for a follow up visit after a car accident. No treatment was performed on the initial visit other than an evaluation and radiographic images on maxillary anterior teeth. What would be an appropriate code for the follow-up visit?

D0170 re-evaluation-limited, problem focused (established patient; not post-operative visit

This descriptor allows for a patient to be seen for an oral evaluation in certain circumstances, including this one where there was a traumatic injury "where no treatment was rendered but patient needs follow-up monitoring."

Summary

The Diagnostic Section of the Code on Dental Procedures and Nomenclature (CDT Code) deals with the gathering of data and cognitive skills necessary for patient evaluation. These 82 codes are the "bread and butter" of the CDT Code and are utilized for every patient throughout the course of care. Attention to detail of descriptors allows for correct coding in treatment, as explained in the scenarios and questions presented in this section. "Coding for what you do" does not mean that all procedures will be covered or reimbursed by third party carriers. However, "coding for what you do" will mean that dental treatment is properly coded and reported, allowing for accuracy and transparency in patient record keeping.

Contributor Biography

Ralph A. Cooley, D.D.S. is a general dentist who was in private practice for more than 30 years and is currently a full time associate professor at the University of Texas School of Dentistry in Houston. He is a past member of the ADA Council on Dental Benefits and is currently a member of the Code Maintenance Committee.

Chapter 2. D1000 – D1999 Preventive

By Paul Reggiardo, D.D.S.

Introduction

Ironically, while the preventive section contains the least number of dental procedure codes, these services are among the most ubiquitously delivered in dentistry for both children and adults. It is thus imperative that offices understand the dental preventive codes and associated dental benefit carrier contract policies that govern third-party reimbursement. Some of these policies for preventive services contain frequency limitations, annual service delivery maximums, age restrictions, and eruption-specific eligibility. While medical necessity and the dentist's judgment of patient benefit must govern all care decisions, the patient has an economic interest in understanding what may constitute a reimbursable preventive service under his or her dental benefit plan. By knowing how individual third-party policies and definitions are applied to preventive dental services, dental professionals can assist patients in best utilizing their dental benefit plans to maintain and optimize oral health.

Another key concept to patient acceptance and appreciation of these services is that preventive is not synonymous with elective. When part of a treatment plan developed by the dentist, each is a necessary and effective component to the preservation or restoration of the patient's oral health. Two services in particular – professionally-applied topical fluoride products and the placement of pit-and-fissure sealants on high caries-risk populations or anatomically caries-susceptible teeth soon after eruption – are widely recognized as positive determinants of future oral health. The failure to provide other preventive services, such as the placement of an appropriate space maintainer to prevent tooth movement and space loss after the extraction or other untimely loss of a primary tooth, has almost immediate harmful consequences.

At a time when patients rightly hold their dental providers accountable for acts of omission, as well as acts of commission, it is crucial that dentists properly diagnose, treatment plan, execute, record and code preventive services with the same clarity, purpose and range as all other treatment categories.

Key Definitions and Concepts

Prophylaxis: Removal of plaque and stains from the tooth structures intended to control local irritational factors.

Prophylaxis is not a therapeutic procedure related to the healing of a disease or condition of the periodontium. These procedures are found under the periodontics codes (D4000-D4999).

The removal of local irritational factors may reduce transitory local gingival inflammation (gingivitis).

Topical application of fluoride varnish and **topical application of fluoride excluding varnish**: Professionally applied prescription topical fluoride products delivered separately from that contained in prophy paste (the mild abrasive compound used usually with rotary cup instrumentation to remove extrinsic stain and dental plaque from the enamel tooth surface).

Sealant: Dental sealants (also known as pit and fissure sealants) are materials placed in anatomically caries-susceptible tooth surfaces (usually posterior occlusal pits and fissures, posterior buccal or lingual pits or grooves, or incisor cingulum pits) after the adjacent tooth structure is mechanically or chemically prepared for enamel bonding. The material, after chemical or light curing, forms a mechanical barrier to the penetration of acid-producing cariogenic bacteria, thereby reducing the potential for caries initiation. The procedure is appropriate prior to dentin cavitation and is most effective when applied to enamel that has not undergone significant enamel demineralization.

Preventive resin restoration in a moderate to high caries risk patient – permanent tooth: Conservative restoration of an active cavitated lesion in a pit or fissure that does not extend into dentin; includes placement of a sealant in any radiating non-carious fissures or pits. This procedure differs from a sealant in that it involves mechanical removal (usually by rotary instrumentation) of demineralized, chalky enamel (enamel caries) and the restoration of the affected tooth surface with a restorative filling material such as a composite resin or glass ionomer cement. Dentin is not penetrated by caries or by instrumentation.

Key Definitions and Concepts

Interim caries arresting medicament application – per tooth: The treatment of an active, non-symptomatic carious lesion by the topical application of a medicament which arrests or inhibits caries progression. It is often (though not exclusively) intended as an interim measure in the medical management of dental caries in selected situations (such as a tooth nearing exfoliation) or populations (such as the frail elderly, the very young, or patients with special healthcare or developmental needs) to stabilize the tooth until it can later be treated in a conventional restorative manner. It is the appropriate code for the application of silver diamine fluoride.

Distal shoe space maintainer – fixed – unilateral: The fabrication and delivery of a fixed space maintaining appliance extending distally and subgingivally from the first primary molar immediately after extraction of the second primary molar to guide the eruption of the unerupted first permanent molar. While technically a type of fixed unilateral space maintainer (D1510), it differs importantly in that it is intended to be removed and replaced with another space maintenance appliance (usually a D1510) upon eruption of the first permanent molar.

Procedure D1510 (space maintainer – fixed, unilateral) specifically excludes the distal shoe space maintainer design.

Changes to This Category

CDT 2019 contains four additions and two deletions to the preventive codes, all having to do with identifying the arch (maxillary or mandibular) in which a bilateral space maintainer is placed. The changes are intended to provide greater specificity to the dental record and to smooth claims processing.

When a bilateral fixed or removable space maintainer is placed, the previous code set was not specific to the arch (maxillary or mandibular) in question. This had in some cases resulted in dental benefit plans delaying payment of the claim in order to obtain arch identification (request for additional information) or, when an appliance was placed in both arches on the same date of service, the second placement was denied as a duplicate entry. The problem also occurred when a second appliance was placed in the opposite arch at a subsequent point in time, and the claim rejected as not meeting the "length of service before replacement" time interval of the policy.

The new codes provide the needed clarity to auto-adjudicate the claim, speed claims processing, lessen the need for additional information requests, and reduce claim rejections.

The two deletions are as follows:

~~**D1515 space maintainer – fixed – bilateral**~~

~~**D1525 space maintainer – removable – bilateral**~~

They are replaced by:

D1516 space maintainer – fixed – bilateral – maxillary

D1517 space maintainer – fixed – bilateral – mandibular

D1526 space maintainer – removable – bilateral – maxillary

D1527 space maintainer – removable – bilateral – mandibular

Diagnosis Codes – ICD-10-CM

The CDT to ICD tables in Appendix 1 provide appropriate guidance on linkages between Preventive procedure codes and diagnosis codes. This chapter does not contain supplemental information on this topic.

Coding Scenarios

CODING SCENARIO #1

Initial Routine Dental Visit of Nine-Year-Old Patient

A new patient, in grade school, is seen for a routine first examination, dental cleaning, and fluoride gel application. No other services or procedures are provided.

How might this visit be coded?

D0150 comprehensive oral evaluation – new or established patient

D1120 prophylaxis – child

D1208 topical application of fluoride – excluding varnish

What if I used a fluoride varnish instead of a fluoride gel?

Then the correct fluoride code would be D1206.

What would change if the patient was 12 years old?

Selection of the prophylaxis code is determined by how the dentist views the patient's dentition. Either the adult (D1110) or the child (D1120) code may be used for patients with transitional dentitions regardless of age. Patient age is not a part of either code's nomenclature or descriptor. ADA policy recommends that dental benefit determinations should be based on dental development rather than patient age. According to the ADA Policy "Age of a Child" adopted in 1991, benefits should be based on stage of dentition:

> "If a plan cannot recognize stage of dentition, age 12 should be recognized as the age of an adult, in terms of dentition (with the exclusion of treatment for orthodontics and sealants)."

The prophylaxis codes are dentition-specific rather than age-specific. Some third-party payers have in their contracts' policies that limit available benefits based on patient age, not stage of dentition. Most of these dental benefit plans specify an age between 12 and 21 as to when the patient is considered an adult.

What if the patient had only permanent teeth with eruption completed through the second permanent molars?

Regardless of age, patients with permanent dentition are appropriately coded using D1110.

What if the patient had eruption completed through the second permanent molars and one or more retained primary tooth or teeth with no succedaneous replacement?

This, then, would represent the patient's full and complete natural permanent dentition and the correct code would be that of the adult prophylaxis (D1110).

CODING SCENARIO #2

Recare Visits After Periodontal Therapy

Following either surgical or non-surgical periodontal therapy the patient is placed by the treating dentist on a program of periodic periodontal maintenance (D4910), which includes removal of bacterial plaque and calculus (mineralized deposits) from subgingival and supragingival tooth surfaces, site-specific scaling and root planning, and coronal tooth polishing. Between these designated periodontal maintenance visits, which continue at varying intervals for the life of the dentition or any implant replacements, the patient is seen by the dentist for routine dental prophylaxis (tooth cleaning procedures).

May the dentist code and bill for this additional procedure (D1110 or D1120) or is this prohibited as a duplication of existing services under D4910?

If the dentist determines that the patient's periodontal health can be augmented with periodic routine prophylaxis procedures (removal of plaque, calculus and stains from the tooth structures for the purpose of controlling local irritational factors), then this service should be performed and reported as D1110 or D1120, depending on the state of the dentition. Nothing in the D4910 or D1110/D11120 code nomenclatures or descriptors make these procedures mutually exclusive.

Does it make any difference if the reporting dentist for prophylaxis (D1110 or D1120) is the same dentist providing periodontal maintenance (D4910)?

No. The dentist should code and report for the services provided regardless of the provision of other services by the same or a different dentist.

Will both procedures be reimbursed by the patient's dental benefit carrier?

Reimbursement will depend upon the dental benefit plan language and the contractual policies governing covered benefits. Regardless of any expected benefit payment, the dentist should provide and code for medically-necessary services that are determined by community standards and the patient's informed consent for these services.

CODING SCENARIO #3

Silver Diamine Fluoride Application

A patient just turned three years old and presents with multiple asymptomatic carious dental lesions involving the maxillary anterior dentition. After consideration of available treatment options and the risks/benefits/alternatives to each approach, the decision is reached by the dentist, in consultation and informed consent with the parent, to utilize a caries arrestment agent (silver diamine fluoride) in a program of medical caries management. Both the dentist and the parent are aware that this procedure (D1354) is not a covered benefit under the patient's dental care plan.

Since silver diamine fluoride is a topical fluoride product, may the dentist code for D1208 (topical application of fluoride – excluding varnish)?

No. The topical application of a prescription fluoride product (gel, rinse, foam or paste delivered without or within a holding tray) for the purpose of enamel remineralization differs from the per tooth application of an agent effective in arresting or inhibiting caries in dentin. The products and the procedures are not interchangeable.

Recognizing the patient is at high caries-risk for the remainder of the dentition not yet exhibiting cavitated lesions, the dentist wishes to apply a topical sodium fluoride varnish (D1206).

May this preventive treatment be provided as a separate billable service on the same day as the application of a caries arresting medicament?

Yes. The two services are not mutually exclusive of each other and are not overlapping codes for the same procedure.

CODING SCENARIO #4

Silver Diamine Fluoride Re-application

Following established protocols and best practice recommendations, the dentist sees the patient four to eight weeks after the initial application and again three months later to assess effectiveness in arresting these carious lesions and to re-apply the silver diamine fluoride.

How might each of these visits be coded?

D0170 re-evaluation – limited, problem focused (established patient; not post-operative visit)

D1354 interim caries arresting medicament application – per tooth

Would these services be considered reimbursable under the patient's dental benefit plan?

Reimbursement by the patient's dental insurance carrier for these services would depend upon the contractual limitations and policies governing covered benefits. Regardless of expected third party payment, the dentist should record and code for the services provided.

Should the dentist charge separately for these additional visits and the services provided, or should the cost be included for a specified time period in the initial application as part of a program of medical caries management?

The decision as to whether a separate fee is made for the services provided on subsequent visits after the initial application of the medicament, and at what intervals these services are provided in addition to the usual routine periodic oral evaluation of the established patient (D0120), is at the discretion of the dentist. No matter what the dentist's billing policy, each specific provided service should be coded and noted in the patient record; when fees are charged the dentist's full fee is entered on the claim.

CODING SCENARIO #5

Silver Diamine Fluoride Therapy for Root Caries

An elderly and frail adult presents to your office with multiple dental root caries and recurrent dental caries along the gingival margins of existing restorations adjacent to receding gingival tissues. You are aware of the efficacy of silver diamine fluoride in treating these lesions, but are unsure how to code for the procedure.

Does the per tooth application of an interim caries arresting medicament (D1354) apply to lesions occurring other than by enamel crown demineralization and secondary dentin exposure and bacterial ingress?

The tooth surface location and etiology of the asymptomatic active carious dental lesion does not change the definition of the service provided by the dentist, which is the application of a treatment agent to arrest or inhibit caries progression. **D1354** is still the correct code for this procedure.

CODING SCENARIO #6

Sealant Repair and Maintenance

An eight-year-old patient in your office received sealants two years ago – you placed them on his first permanent molars shortly after his sixth birthday. Today on his routine preventive care (recall) visit, you note partial sealant loss on the mandibular right first permanent molar. The remaining sealant is not easily dislodged with an explorer and you are confident about the integrity of the residual marginal bond. You elect to replace the missing sealant material.

What is the proper code for this procedure?

Because you are not removing the remaining sealant material and are replacing only that which has been lost, you are accomplishing procedure **D1353 (sealant repair – per tooth)**. If, instead, you had removed all residual sealant material and placed a completely new sealant across all occlusal pits, grooves and fissures you would be performing procedure **D1351 (sealant – per tooth)**.

Would either procedure be reimbursable service under the patient's dental benefit plan?

As with all other services, this would depend on benefit plan restrictions and limitations, such as time intervals after initial placement or if replacements are a benefit. Regardless, the dentist must code for the specific service provided.

CODING SCENARIO #7

Removal and Replacement of a Fixed Space Maintainer

A seven-year-old patient of record for whom you previously placed two band-and-loop design fixed unilateral space maintainers (D1510) is scheduled by his neurologist for MRI imaging of a suspected benign tumor of the brain. His neurologist requests the removal of the two space maintainers. Accordingly, you see the patient on two occasions: one to remove the appliances before the procedure and the other to re-cement or re-bond after the procedure.

How could these visits be coded?

Appliance Removal Visit

D9999 unspecified adjunctive procedure, by report

This is a more accurate depiction and one which would require that a description of this unusual service be included in the patient record and on any third-party billing.

Note: **D1555** (removal of a fixed space maintainer) is **not** appropriate in this scenario because the descriptor limits this procedure to a "dentist or practice that did not originally place the appliance."

Appliance Replacement Visit

D1550 re-cement or re-bond space maintainer is the appropriate and accurate coding for this service, which does not exclude any provider class.

CODING SCENARIO #8

Procedures for the Placement of a Fixed Space Maintainer

Following the loss of the mandibular right first and second primary molars to dentoalveolar abscess at six years of age, the dentist elects to place a fixed bilateral space maintainer (lingual holding arch) soldered to bands cemented on the fully-erupted first permanent molars. This requires two visits: the first to size the bands and obtain an impression of the arch and the second to deliver and cement into place the fabricated appliance.

The dentist would prefer to post the fee for the appliance at the time the impression is taken and casts sent to the dental laboratory for appliance fabrication. The dental benefit carrier demands that charges be posted only after delivery of the appliance. Which should prevail?

Historically, the dentist has preferred to post the cost of the service at the time of tooth preparation in the case of indirect restorations or at the time of impression in the case of dental appliances. Likewise third-party payers adjudicate claims and make reimbursements based on the dental benefit plan coverage provisions. What prevails are the legally enforceable provisions of the dental benefit plan and the provisions of an applicable participating provider agreement.

Coding Q&A

1. What is the definition of prophylaxis?

A prophylaxis is removal of plaque, calculus and stains from the tooth structures. It is intended to control local irritational factors. It is a preventive and not a therapeutic procedure.

2. Does the patient's age dictate whether a child or adult prophylaxis is reported?

The prophylaxis codes are dentition specific rather than age specific and should be reported in this manner. However, some third-party payers may have restrictions in their contracts that limit available benefits or benefit levels based on age and not stage of the dentition. The ADA House of Delegates in 1991 adopted a policy (Age of Child (1991:635)) concerning this issue that:

- Benefits should be based on the stage of the dentition
- If a plan cannot recognize the stage of the dentition, age 12 should be recognized as the age of an adult (with the exclusion of treatment for orthodontics and sealants).

Nonetheless, prophylaxis claims may be rejected by third-party carriers as not meeting plan age specifications for this service. For patients with transitional dentition the claim may be submitted as either a child or adult prophylaxis, as the transitional dentition is included in both codes. For patients exhibiting an adult dentition (adult tooth eruption completed through the second permanent molars), the claim may need to be appealed.

3. What code is appropriate for a difficult prophylaxis?

There is no separate procedure code that reflects a greater degree of difficulty of a dental prophylaxis. The available prophylaxis codes are "D1110 prophylaxis - adult" and "D1120 prophylaxis - child."

However, if the patient's clinical condition reveals moderate to severe gingival inflammation without bone loss, it may be that this should not be considered a "difficult prophy" scenario. Rather, the patient's condition may more appropriately be treated by the D4346 procedure.

4. **When might a patient have benefits coverage for more than the usual two prophylaxis procedures in a 12-month period or in a calendar year?**

   Some dental benefit plans may allow more frequent prophylaxis procedures based on medical risk or other factors (e.g., diabetic/immuno suppressed; pregnancy).

   Other patients in the same plan who are not deemed "at risk" would be subject to standard frequency limitations. If the dentist determines medical necessity for more frequent cleanings not provided under plan parameters, the dentist or the patient may explore the plan's appeal process or that appeal process provided under state regulation.

5. **What code is used to report a scaling and root planing in the presence of generalized moderate or severe gingival inflammation?**

   When the dentist's oral evaluation determines that any inflammation present is localized and there is no loss of attachment or bone, a prophylaxis procedure is appropriate and would be reported with the applicable CDT code (D1110 or D1120). Should, however, the evaluation reveal generalized moderate to severe gingival inflammation, again with no loss of attachment or bone, the scaling procedure D4346 is instead appropriate. **D4346 (scaling in the presence of generalized moderate or severe gingival inflammation – full mouth, after oral evaluation)** should be provided and reported as a separate procedure and not in conjunction with prophylaxis.

6. **After a full mouth gross debridement (D4355) for the purpose of enabling a later comprehensive periodontal evaluation is delivered, may the patient receive a prophylaxis procedure on the next visit?**

   A dental prophylaxis (cleaning) may be delivered on the next visit, if indicated. The appropriate sequence of services would be D4355 followed after an appropriate interval, by an oral evaluation. The oral evaluation findings may indicate that a prophylaxis is the next appropriate periodontal service.

7. **Can "D1110 prophylaxis – adult" and "D4342 scaling and root planing – one to three teeth per quadrant" be reported on the same date of service?**

   There is no language in the descriptor of an adult prophylaxis that precludes the reporting of any other procedure on the same date of service and no language in the descriptor of D4342 which precludes at the same visit the provision of a dental prophylaxis. However, third party reimbursement for these procedures is dependent on the specific dental benefit plan provisions. Some plans may pay for both services when delivered at the same time, while others might impose a specified interval.

8. **Could the CDT code D1206 (topical application of fluoride varnish) be used when applying fluoride varnish to desensitize a tooth?**

   No. When fluoride varnish is utilized to desensitize a tooth, the appropriate CDT code is **D9910 application of desensitizing medicament**. CDT code **D1206 application of topical fluoride varnish** is exclusive to the use for caries prevention.

9. **If a dental office uses fluoride varnish as part of its recall visit protocol, should it continue to report codes D1203 or D1204 as it has done in the past, or should it use a newer fluoride varnish code?**

   On January 1, 2013, the CDT Code set eliminated separate topical fluoride application codes (D1203 and D1204) for children and for adults. All professional topical fluoride applications for both adults and children are now documented using D1208 application of topical fluoride – excluding varnish or D1206 topical application of fluoride varnish. Fluoride materials that are not considered varnish include gels, foams, or aqueous solutions.

10. **When resin is applied to a tooth's pit and fissure area, what distinguishes a sealant (D1351) from a preventive resin restoration (D1352)?**

    The CDT Code was revised effective January 1, 2011, to enable separate reporting of these distinct procedures. Application of an unfiled resin or glass ionomer cement limited to the enamel surface is a sealant procedure and would be documented using **D1351**. When a filled resin or glass ionomer cement is applied to an area of an active cavitated lesion that does not extend into the dentin, this procedure is a preventive resin restoration and the applicable procedure code is **D1352**.

    Note: Should the lesion extend into the dentin, the procedure code for a one surface composite resin restoration (**D2391**) would be used to document the service.

11. **Sometimes dental sealants fail completely (i.e., no sealant material remains bonded to the tooth surface), but most often failure is incremental with a partial loss of sealant material. The fix is to reapply sealant material only to the unprotected caries-susceptible pits and fissures. This is a much more limited procedure than D1351, which applies when the entire tooth surface is re-sealed. What CDT code applies to a sealant repair?**

    In the past, the sealant repair procedure was documented with "D1999 unspecified preventive procedure, by report." The CDT code D1353 (sealant repair per tooth) now fills this coding gap.

Summary

The 21 codes which comprise the preventive section are thankfully straightforward and easy to understand because some of these procedures are among the most common services in dental practice, especially in the care of infants and children. Prevention of dental disease is the cornerstone of the profession and procedures such as professional removal plaque and calculus, application of prescription strength topical fluoride, nutritional counseling, oral hygiene instruction, and sealant placement help ensure optimal oral health.

Contributor Biography

Paul Reggiardo, D.D.S. is a practicing pediatric dentist in Huntington Beach, California, and a Clinical Assistant Professor of the Division of Dental Public Health and Pediatric Dentistry at the Herman Ostrow School of Dentistry of the University of Southern California. He serves as chair of the American Academy of Pediatric Dentistry Committee on Dental Benefit Programs and is a voting member of the American Dental Association's Code Maintenance Committee, representing the AAPD.

Chapter 3.
D2000 – D2999 Restorative

By Fred L. Horowitz, D.M.D.

Introduction

Restorative codes continue to represent the majority of dental procedures done in a general dental practice on a day-to-day basis. Selection of the applicable code, or codes, for restorative services is generally straightforward when the user understands the CDT Code's underlying organization and concepts. However, the advent of new technology can present some challenges.

In this chapter, some basic terms are defined, recent restorative code changes are discussed, use is illustrated in common coding scenarios, and it concludes with several FAQ. Some new examples have been added in the FAQ section to help the practitioner best apply the codes to the procedures performed.

Key Definitions and Concepts

Direct Restorations

Amalgam restorations include the tooth preparation, all adhesives (including amalgam bonding agents), as well as liners and bases. If pins are used, they are reported separately using the applicable procedure code (see D2951).

The amalgam codes are used to report procedures performed on primary or permanent dentition, with no differentiation between anterior and posterior teeth.

Resin-based composite restorations include tooth preparation, acid etching, adhesives, liners and bases and curing of the material. If pins are used, they are reported separately (see D2951.) There is no differentiation based on the various composite resin materials utilized.

The resin-based composite codes are used for reporting procedures performed on the primary or permanent dentition. However, unlike amalgam codes the resin-based codes differentiate between procedures performed on anterior and posterior dentition.

All **glass ionomers**, when used as restorations, are reported using the resin-based composite codes.

Indirect Restorations

Inlay restorations are intra-coronal restorations made outside the mouth. They conform to a prepared cavity and do not restore any cusp tips.

Onlay restorations are made outside the mouth. They cover one or more cusp tips and adjoining occlusal surfaces, but not the entire external surface.

Crown restorations are made outside the mouth. They cover all of the cusps on posterior teeth, extend beyond the height of contour on all covered surfaces and restore all four proximal surfaces.

¾ crown restorations are made outside the mouth. They cover all of the cusps on posterior teeth, extend beyond the height of contour on the covered surfaces and restore three of the four proximal surfaces.

Explanation of Restorations

This table was updated in CDT 2017 to clarify that "Facial" and "Labial" are synonymous when describing surfaces involved in a restoration.

Location	Number of Surfaces	Characteristics
Anterior	1	Placed on one of the following five surface classifications – Mesial, Distal, Incisal, Lingual, or Facial (or Labial)
	2	Placed, without interruption, on two of the five surface classifications – e.g., Mesial-Lingual
	3	Placed, without interruption, on three of the five surface classifications – e.g., Lingual-Mesial-Facial (or Labial)
	4 or more	Placed, without interruption, on four or more of the five surface classifications – e.g., Mesial-Incisal-Lingual-Facial (or Labial)
Posterior	1	Placed on one of the following five surface classifications – Mesial, Distal, Occlusal, Lingual, or Buccal
	2	Placed, without interruption, on two of the five surface classifications – e.g., Mesial-Occlusal
	3	Placed, without interruption, on three of the five surface classifications – e.g., Lingual-Occlusal-Distal
	4 or more	Placed, without interruption, on four or more of the five surface classifications – e.g., Mesial-Occlusal-Lingual-Distal

Note: Tooth surfaces are reported on the HIPAA standard electronic dental transaction and the ADA Dental Claim Form using the letters in the following table.

Surface	Code
Buccal	B
Distal	D
Facial (or Labial)	F
Incisal	I
Lingual	L
Mesial	M
Occlusal	O

Changes to This Category

There are no additions, revisions, deletions or editorial changes for this category in CDT 2019.

Diagnosis Codes – ICD-10-CM

The CDT to ICD tables in Appendix 1 provide appropriate guidance on linkages between Restorative procedure codes and diagnosis codes. This chapter does not contain supplemental information on this topic.

ICD codes are used to indicate a diagnosis, observation or finding. The relationship between ICD and CDT codes presented are a partial listing of potential procedures (CDT) that could be utilized to address such diagnosis, findings or observations. They are not meant to be all inclusive, and may be modified as technology and outcomes dictate.

Coding Scenarios

CODING SCENARIO #1

Fractured Tooth – After Hours Visit and the Final Restoration

The patient presents with a broken front tooth on Saturday, a day the office was usually closed. On examination, tooth #8 appeared to have a fractured mesial-incisal angle and lost a mesial composite restoration, with no pain reported. The doctor removed enough tooth structure to fit and cement a polycarbonate crown. The patient was told that the tooth would need a porcelain-fused-to-metal crown (PFM), but this could be done at a scheduled appointment during regular office hours.

How could you code for this after hours visit?

D0140 limited oral evaluation – problem focused

D2799 provisional crown – further treatment or completion of diagnosis necessary prior to final impression

Note: D2799 is used instead of **D2970 temporary crown (fractured tooth)** because D2970 was deleted as of CDT 2016. The Code Maintenance Committee determined that the entry was limiting by specifying "fractured tooth" in the nomenclature, and there are other codes that more accurately describe the procedure and its intended outcome (i.e., **D2799 provisional crown** or **D2940 protective restoration**).

D9440 office visit – after regularly scheduled hours

Note: The after-hours office visit code (**D9440**) is from the Adjunctive Services section of the Code and can be reported in addition to the other services performed at that appointment. This service may not be covered or reimbursed by some dental benefits plans.

When the patient returned to the office, the doctor removes the polycarbonate crown. Following caries excavation, the doctor determines that the tooth required some replacement of lost structure to achieve proper strength and retention for the crown. One threaded titanium pin and a bonded resin core material were used to restore the tooth, followed by a preparation and an impression for a PFM. The PFM was fabricated using an alloy containing gold 15%, Palladium 25 % and Platinum 10%.

How would this visit during regular office hours be coded?

D2950 core buildup, including any pins, when required

Replacement of tooth structure that is more than simply filling undercuts is appropriately reported using the code for a core buildup (**D2950**). The retentive pin that was placed is included in the procedure documented with this code.

Note: D2950 would not be appropriate if the material is used only to eliminate undercuts or to yield a more ideal form for a subsequent indirect restoration. In this situation the procedure would be documented as "D2949 restorative foundation for an indirect restoration."

D2752 crown – porcelain fused to noble metal

The code for a PFM utilizing a noble metal (**D2752**) rather than a high noble metal (**D2750**) was selected because the alloy used in the crown contains more than 25% but less than 60% noble metals.

CODING SCENARIO #2

Indirect Restorations – Laboratory Crowns vs. In-Office

CAD/CAM crowns

Doctor A has a CAD/CAM in his office. It is now being used to mill an esthetic post and core for tooth #8. When completed, the post and core is cemented and the tooth prepared for the final all-ceramic crown. The crown is milled with the same machine.

Doctor B uses a dental lab to prepare crowns. Today's treatment involves restoring #8 with a fine cast gold post and core created from an impression taken at the patient's prior visit. After cementing the cast post and core the dentist will take the final impression for a porcelain jacket crown which would be fabricated using a traditional porcelain layering technique by the dental lab.

What CDT codes are appropriate for these procedures?

Doctor A and Doctor B use the same CDT codes.

D2952 post and core indirectly fabricated – in addition to crown

Although Doctor A did not take an impression, the milled post and core was custom fabricated using an indirect method. Since casting metal posts and cores is also an indirect method, **D2952** continues to be the correct code for Doctor B's procedure.

D2740 crown – porcelain/ceramic

An all ceramic crown, whether milled or built up and vacuum-fired, is coded using **D2740**.

CODING SCENARIO #3

Multiple Restorations on the Same Tooth

Visit #1

Patient presents with braces, radiographs acquired by the orthodontist, and evidence of poor oral hygiene. Radiographs show dark triangles just below the contact between nearly every posterior tooth, evidence of incipient decay. Immediate treatment was fluoride varnish application to teeth that may be conserved, and the following composite resin restorations – #14, separate MO and DO; #19, an MOD and a buccal pit restoration.

How would you code for the procedures on this first visit?

D1206 topical application of fluoride varnish

Fluoride varnish was applied and application of this material has its own code.

D2392 resin-based composite – two surface, posterior

D2392 is applicable to #14 which had separate two-surface restorations; report twice, once for the MO and the second for the DO.

D2393 resin-based composite – three surface, posterior

D2391 resin-based composite – one surface, posterior

Both are applicable to #19; report D2393 for the MOD and D2391 for the buccal pit restoration.

Note: Dental plans may have clauses that restrict coverage on the same surface twice on the same date of service, and an alternate benefit provision may be applied. For example, payers often downcode separate restorations by recoding them as a single multiple surface restoration. Nevertheless, when individual restorations on the same teeth are done, they should be reported separately. Remember "Code for what you do."

Visit #2

Patient presents with an area of decayed enamel on the buccal surface of #28, below where the bracket had been bonded. The doctor removed the caries and demineralized enamel without penetrating into the dentin. Composite resin was used to restore the cavity.

How would you code for the procedure on the second visit?

An orthodontic patient with brackets is considered one with high caries risk. Since the resin restoration placed did not extend into the dentin, the applicable CDT code is:

D1352 preventive resin restoration in a moderate to high risk caries risk patient – permanent tooth

Note: Should this restoration be place on a primary tooth, the applicable code is:

D2999 unspecified restorative procedure, by report

CODING SCENARIO #4

Modifying an Existing Partial Denture After an Extraction

The patient presented complaining that he could not wear his upper partial because of some loose, painful teeth. After visual inspection the doctor determined that a well-designed maxillary removable partial denture had been placed and that it could be reused. This partial replaced teeth #2, 3, 4, and 14, with clasps on teeth #5, 13, and 15. The doctor's examination indicated that tooth #13 had Class III mobility due to advanced periodontal bone loss; #12 was fractured and decayed so that only a small piece of root remained exposed; and #15 had a fractured MOBL silver amalgam restoration with a fair amount of recurrent decay.

These findings led to a treatment plan that contained several separate procedures, coded as follows:

Extraction of teeth #12 and #13

D7140 extraction, erupted tooth or exposed root (elevation and/or forceps removal)

Both the routine extraction of #13 and the root tip removal of #12 could be coded using **D7140**. If the root tip removal required the laying of a mucoperiosteal flap and bone removal, the appropriate code for surgical extractions is **D7210**.

Addition of teeth #12 and #13 to the partial

D5650 add tooth to existing partial denture

This procedure is reported twice in this scenario, one time for each tooth added, and generally requires reporting the tooth number added (based on its anatomy).

Additional clasp to the partial for retention on tooth #11

D5660 add clasp to existing partial denture – per tooth

There is a single code for the addition of a clasp to a partial, whether it is wrought wire and processed or cast and soldered.

Full cast noble metal crown (tooth #15) to fit the existing clasp

D2792 crown – full cast noble metal

D2971 additional procedures to construct new crown under existing partial denture framework

When a crown is constructed to fit an existing partial denture the code for a regular crown is selected based on the material from which it is fabricated. The additional procedures required to allow the crown to accommodate the existing clasp are coded using **D2971**.

CODING SCENARIO #5

A Child Who Needs Endodontic Treatment and a Crown

It was a sad story that the doctor had heard too often. The three-year-old patient had early childhood caries and was in pain. Treatment consisted of three pulpectomies followed by a resorbable filling and four esthetic-coated stainless steel crowns cemented on the maxillary incisors.

How would you code for this encounter?

Endodontic procedure

D3230 pulpal therapy (resorbable filling)-anterior, primary tooth (excluding final restoration)

"Pulpal therapy" with a resorbable filling is a typical pulp treatment for primary teeth that have carious pulp exposure. It is reported three times in this case, once for each treated tooth.

Primary crowns

D2934 prefabricated esthetic coated stainless steel crown – primary tooth

There are three types of stainless steel crowns for primary teeth: the standard stainless steel crown, one with a resin window and the esthetic coated stainless steel crown. The esthetic coated crown was used in this case and it is reported four times on the claim.

CODING SCENARIO #6

Treating Acute Pulpitis

The patient's diagnosis was acute pulpitis of tooth #5. During the first appointment, the dentist opened tooth #5 to gain access to the pulp chamber and removed the tissue with a broach. Tooth closure was a temporary filling.

Ten days later the patient returned to have the root canal completed. The canal was opened, thoroughly flushed and cleaned, then obturated with gutta percha and an appropriate sealer.

What codes are applicable to the endodontic treatment on each appointment?

Visit #1

D3221 pulpal debridement

D2940 protective restoration

These procedures describe the simple removal of acutely inflamed pulp tissue and closure with a temporary restoration, for the relief of pain. This is not a definitive endodontic treatment.

Visit #2

D3320 endodontic therapy, premolar tooth (excluding final restoration)

This is a completed root canal therapy using an appropriate endodontic therapy procedure code.

Note: Language in the descriptor of **D3221** pulpal debridement precludes the same provider from reporting this procedure on the same date as an endodontic therapy (**D3320**) procedure. Since the date of completion of the root canal is different from the date of initiation of the procedure, and the patient presented with an emergency, both codes may be reported.

CODING SCENARIO #7

Failed Endodontically Treated Tooth with Post, Core and Crown

The patient complained of "a bad taste in their mouth" at a routine recall exam and prophylaxis. Upon examination the doctor found a draining fistula between teeth #28 and #29. After reviewing the chart and taking a periapical radiographic image, the doctor determined that #28 root canal therapy was failing. Additionally, there was decay evident at the distal margin of the PFM crown.

How would you code to treat this situation?

D1110 prophylaxis – adult
D0120 periodic oral evaluation – established patient
D0220 intraoral – periapical first radiographic image
D2955 post removal
D3347 retreatment of previous root canal therapy – bicuspid
D2954 prefabricated post and core in addition to crown
D2740 crown – porcelain/ceramic

CODING SCENARIO #8

Patient with Fractured Tooth and Uncertain Diagnosis

A patient comes to the dental office at the end of the day, presenting with a fractured clinical crown that occurred earlier that same day. The tooth is somewhat sensitive to cold, and there appears to be a potential horizontal fracture of the root 5mm below the crestal bone. But you cannot determine that definitively. There are no other symptoms. The decision is made to fabricate a provisional crown and re-evaluate at a later date or sooner if symptoms intensify or new symptoms develop.

How would you code to treat this situation?

D2799 provisional crown

As no definitive diagnosis can be made, nor final restoration prepared, you would not categorize this as a temporary crown made during the fabrication of a permanent restoration (crown).

1. **How may I document and report local anesthesia as a separate procedure when restorative (or any other operative or surgical) services are being delivered?**

   D9215 local anesthesia in conjunction with operative or surgical procedures is the available code if you wish to document and report this procedure separately. Benefit plan limitations may preclude separate reimbursement for local anesthesia.

2. **I know there are no differences between primary teeth and permanent teeth for most indirect restorations. Are there direct restorative codes for primary teeth?**

   The codes listed for direct restorative procedures are applicable for treatment of primary or permanent dentition.

3. **How do I report two separate two-surface restorations on the same tooth? Carriers advise me to report a MO amalgam and a DO amalgam as a MOD restoration. Is this correct?**

   The carriers' advice is incorrect. Dentists must document the procedures performed, and reporting these restorations separately as a MO and a DO is appropriate. Following the carriers' advice would likely lead to a discrepancy between your records for the patient and the claim submission, which is a bad situation.

   Note: Some dental plans may have clauses that restrict coverage on the same surface twice on the same date of service. This is why the carriers may apply an alternate benefit provision that leads to reimbursement of the two separate 2-surface restorations as a single 3-surface restoration.

4. **I recently purchased a laser and have been unable to find any "laser" codes in the Code on Dental Procedures and Nomenclature.**

   The codes are procedure based rather than instrument based. You would report the appropriate code based on the actual procedure that was performed.

5. **What code do I report for an incisal restoration?**

   If the restoration involves the incisal angle, code **D2335 resin-based composite – four or more surfaces or involving incisal angle (anterior)** may be reported. If the incisal surface restored does not involve the incisal angle, report with the appropriate anterior procedure code that describes the number of surfaces restored.

6. **Should single crowns that are splinted together be coded as single crowns (in the D27xx series of codes) or as a bridge (in the D67xx series)?**

   Single crowns that are splinted together are appropriately reported as single crowns, D27xx. There is no coding mechanism to report splinting the crowns.

   Note: Prosthodontic retainers are parts of a fixed partial denture that attach a pontic to the abutment tooth, implant abutment, or implant and should be used in conjunction with a pontic code.

7. **What procedure code should I report for a porcelain fused to a zirconium substrate crown?**

   This question contains a commonly made error, using the word zirconium when describing the crown's material. Dental crowns use zirconia, which is an oxide and considered chemically to be a ceramic.

   With this in mind, the applicable procedure code is **D2740 crown – porcelain/ceramic**.

8. **How do I code a porcelain fused to titanium crown? I only see a code for titanium code "D2794 crown – titanium."**

   D2974 is the only crown procedure code that includes "titanium" in its nomenclature, and was intended to apply to any type of crown that contained this metal. The alternative would be to report delivery of a porcelain fused to titanium crown with D2999 unspecified restorative procedure, by report.

9. **Is there a code for retrofitting a new crown to an existing partial denture?**

   The code is **D2971 additional procedures to construct new crown under existing partial denture framework** and should be reported in addition to the crown.

10. **Is there a procedure code for re-cementing an onlay?**

    D2910 re-cement or re-bond inlay, onlay, or partial coverage restoration includes the re-cementation of an onlay, as well as inlays and any other partial coverage restorations such as a veneer.

11. **If I place an IRM (intermediate restorative material) restoration, do I report this as sedative restoration or a palliative procedure?**

    Delivery and reporting a protective restoration (D2940) or palliative (e.g., emergency) treatment of dental pain (D9110) is based on the dentist's clinical judgment. However, both codes would not be reported simultaneously for the same procedure on the same date of service.

12. **With all the restorative codes published in the CDT manual, when may it be necessary to consider using "D2999 unspecified restorative procedure, by report" to document and report services rendered?**

    No matter how many definitive CDT codes exist exceptional situations arise, sometimes due to widespread adoption of a new procedure, the CDT Code's maintenance timetable, or due to limited frequency or scope of occurrence. Some examples of situations where D2999 would be applicable follow:

    - The restorative procedure was started but was not completed due to clinical complications requiring a referral (e.g., extensive decay necessitating surgical extraction instead of direct restoration) or patient compliance (e.g., patient does not return for placement of permanent crown).
    - The patient's treatment plan includes placement of a prefabricated post and core under an existing crown.
    - The patient's treatment plan includes placement of a prefabricated post without a core.

13. An access cavity was made through a crown for endodontic treatment. What procedure code is appropriate to report sealing an endodontic access cavity?

There is no code that specifically refers to placement of a restoration to seal an endodontic access cavity. Sealing the access cavity is a procedure reported with the appropriate direct restoration code.

14. I placed a temporary restoration to protect my patient's tooth structure and surrounding tissues. Would "D2940 protective restoration" be appropriate for reporting this procedure?

Yes, D2940 is appropriate based on the code's descriptor, which follows:

Direct placement of a restorative material to protect tooth and/or tissue form. This procedure may be used to relieve pain, promote healing, or prevent further deterioration. Not to be used for endodontic access closure, or as a base or liner under restoration.

15. There are post and core codes only in the restorative category, but not in the fixed prosthodontics category. What is the correct code to use when the final restoration will be a multiple unit fixed bridge?

The codes in the restorative category may be used when a single crown or a multiple unit fixed prosthesis is the final restoration. Remember the placement of codes within categories is to enable ease of navigation through the CDT Code and does not limit use of codes across specialties:

D2952 post and core in addition to crown, indirectly fabricated

D2954 prefabricated post and core in addition to crown

16. **What code should be reported for placement of a composite restoration in a non-carious cervical lesion or an erosive lesion in a cusp tip or other surface of a tooth?**

    Such lesions are treated with resin materials, which include glass ionomers, and the appropriate code depends on tooth position: anterior or posterior. The applicable code for an anterior tooth is:

    D2330 resin-based composite – one surface, anterior

    For a posterior tooth the applicable code is:

    D2391 resin-based composite – one surface, posterior
    Used to restore a carious lesion into the dentin or a deeply eroded area into the dentin. Not a preventive procedure.

    Note: Non-carious cervical lesions commonly extend into the dentin due to thin enamel at this portion of a tooth's anatomy. In an exceptional situation where the lesion does not extend into a posterior tooth's dentin the available procedure code is:

    D2999 unspecified restorative procedure, by report

17. **I repaired a porcelain "chip" on a PFM crown. What procedure code would I use?**

    D2980 crown repair necessitated by restorative material failure

18. **A college student presented with a "chip" on #10. The patient had an enamel fracture of the disto-incisal of #10. She had the chipped piece of enamel. I bonded the fractured enamel piece back on the tooth until the patient could get back to her hometown dentist. What procedure code should I use?**

    D2921 reattachment of tooth fragment, incisal edge or cusp

19. A child became uncooperative as I was removing the decay on a primary molar. I was able to remove all the decay but unable to place a permanent restoration due to the patient's behavior. Eventually the primary molar will need a stainless steel crown. However the patient needs more caries control prior to definitive treatment. How should I code this?

    D2941 interim therapeutic restoration – primary dentition

20. I had to remove a post and core on tooth #9. What code should I use to document this?

    D2955 post removal

21. The periodontal diagnosis suggests the fabrication of two adjacent single crowns that are splinted for additional strength to oppose masticatory forces. Appropriate individual crown codes should be utilized, as there is no CDT coding mechanism to indicate the crowns are splinted. How should I code this?

    D2750 porcelain fused to high noble metal

    This procedure is reported twice, and the patient's record should note that the individual crowns were splinted for additional strength. The splint may be reported with D2999 unspecified restorative procedure, by report.

    On future visits, an ICD-10 code of Z98.811 can be used to indicate dental restoration status.

22. A patient presented with a fractured gold inlay. The doctor placed a provisional inlay, anticipating a final restoration. What code should be used to report this treatment?

    D2999 unspecified restorative procedure, by report

23. A patient presented with a partial fracture of a fixed partial denture. The doctor believes this can be repaired without complete replacement. What code should be used to report the repair?

    D6980 fixed partial denture repair necessitated by restorative material failure

Summary

Restorative procedures are an integral part of treatment that patients receive every day. Because we use the restorative codes so frequently, we must make sure that over time we are indeed using the correct code. It is important for the dentist and the coder to be familiar with any CDT Code changes that enable them to more accurately document and report the procedure delivered to a patient.

Remember, "Code for what you do and do what you code for."

Contributor Biography

Fred L. Horowitz, D.M.D. is president of Primecare Benefits, Inc. a dental insurance holding company based in Nevada. Following graduation from Washington University School of Dental Medicine, Dr Horowitz completed a general practice residency at Sinai Hospital of Detroit. He practiced full time for ten years and has since had executive level positions with dental benefits companies across the country. He is also a three-term board member of the National Association of Dental Plans (NADP), and served on the Board of the National Dental EDI Council, and the National Association of Specialty Health Organizations. He represented the United States dental payer industry to the International Health Terminology Standards Development Organization (now SNOMED), serving as the Vice-Chairman of the International Dental SIG component. He also currently serves on the Joint Operating Committee of the Culinary Health Center.

Chapter 4.
D3000 – D3999 Endodontics

By Kenneth Wiltbank, D.D.S.

Introduction

Endodontics utilizes the 3000 section of the CDT Code. These codes concern procedures related to maintenance of the pulp, regeneration of the pulp and, of course, removal of the pulp and obturating the space where it previously existed. There are surgical codes that pertain to endodontics, including periradicular surgeries as well as use of bone grafting and bone regenerating materials.

Some of the main challenges and questions that are typical to endodontics involve how to code for procedures when they are done in more than one appointment. Other frequently asked questions deal with what things are considered a part of the root canal and what things can be coded separately, such as when to use codes D3331 (root canal obstruction) or D9630 (drugs dispensed in the office) for special endodontic irrigation at home in conjunction with a root canal code in the claim. Another example would be the question of which radiographs are a part of the root canal procedure and which can be separately coded. Separately, CDT Code entries for procedures that involve pulpal regeneration are clear, but they are less commonly used and can be confusing unless the process has been studied by the office coding specialist.

Key Definitions and Concepts

Root canal: This term is used both for the anatomical space where the pulp and blood vessels reside in a vital tooth, and to describe a procedure done to evacuate, clean and fill that same space with a dental material. Thus, it has two different definitions as a noun, and is also occasionally used as a verb: "to root canal." Some teeth have a single root canal space, while others have several root canal spaces. A root canal procedure for a given tooth treats all of the root canal spaces in that tooth.

Pulpectomy: The process wherein a dentist removes the nerve entirely from the root canal space. This process varies in difficulty, tooth by tooth.

Pulpotomy: The process wherein a dentist removes the pulp from the pulp chamber but not the root canal spaces in a tooth. Can be used as a temporary solution to relieve symptoms, or as a permanent solution for a tooth likely to be able to maintain vital pulp in its roots, despite impingement upon the pulp in the pulp chamber.

Irrigation: Part of the pulpectomy where a fluid is used to flush out the canal while cleaning the canal. A standard part of the root canal procedure.

Obturate: The process of filling the space where the nerve used to reside, with some type of dental material. This process must be complete in order to claim that the root canal is finished. After obturation, the tooth will still need final, coronal restoration.

Dental dam: A part of the root canal procedure wherein a tooth is isolated by clamping around it and placing a flexible, tight, rubber-like sheet that will keep the equipment and irrigants on the dentist's side and a patient's saliva on the other side, away from the pulp chamber that is being kept sterile. Dams are considered standard operating procedure per the American Association of Endodontist's Position Statement entitled, "Dental Dams" found at:

> *www.aae.org/specialty/wp-content/uploads/sites/2/2017/06/dentaldamstatement.pdf*

There are some root canal treatments where extraordinary measures have to be taken to fit a dental dam over a tooth. In these cases dam placement is documented using CDT code **D3910 surgical procedure for isolation of tooth with rubber dam**.

Pulpal regeneration: A procedure, likely to include multiple appointments, whose intention is to sterilize a root canal space, then encourage vital tissue to grow back into that canal space in an attempt to strengthen a weak tooth and regain vital tissue in the pulp canal space..

Apexification: A procedure traditionally used to treat similar types of teeth as pulpal regeneration. In these cases, multiple appointments are used in a tooth that became necrotic, to develop a "stop" at its root end, that can allow a better obturation of its root.

Apexogenesis: A procedure similar to pulpotomy, but often less aggressive. The purpose being, to allow pulp to continue to exist and thrive in the pulp chamber and root canal space below.

Changes to This Category

There were no changes to this category in CDT 2019.

Diagnosis Codes – ICD-10-CM

The CDT to ICD tables in Appendix 1 provide appropriate guidance on linkages between Endodontics procedure codes and diagnosis codes.

Note: Claims against medical benefit plans use the AMA's CPT code set to report procedures, and the ICD code set for diagnoses. There are two main situations in which endodontists would use CPT codes and corresponding ICD-10 codes:

- Trauma cases, where a medical insurance plan has been assigned to cover expenses of the accident
- When dental benefit plan provisions require surgical codes be submitted through medical insurance prior to being submitted for dental benefits

There are several CDT codes used to document procedures delivered for an endodontic case that have comparable CPT codes:

- Diagnostics – D0140-D0171 correspond to CPT codes 99201-99204 for new patients, and 99212-99215 for established patients.
- Radiographs – D0220 and D0230 correspond to CPT codes 70300 and 70310, respectively.
- Endodontic procedures – D3000-D3999 correspond to the single CPT code 41899 that is defined as "unlisted procedure, dentoalveolar structure."

CODING SCENARIO #1

Root Canal Started in Another State

A patient presents to a dental office having had a root canal started on a single rooted tooth #29 in another state while on vacation. The patient is not in any pain. An exam is performed and a diagnostic, preoperative radiograph is made and evaluated. The radiograph shows evidence of a large periapical radiolucency as well as radiopaque evidence that calcium hydroxide has likely been placed in the root canal space. A treatment plan is made so that the patient might have the root canal completed, a buildup is placed and a crown made.

At the appointment in which the root canal is intended to be completed, it is found that ninety minutes was insufficient to complete the case and as well, and surprisingly, a significant amount of purulent exudate came into the tooth from the periapical tissues. A second appointment was made.

During the second appointment, the root canal was completed to a good result and a buildup was placed. An intraoperative radiograph and two post-operative radiographs were made during this appointment. A crown preparation appointment was made.

What procedure codes would be used to document and report the services provided during each of the three encounters?

Visit #1 (patient presents)

D0140 limited exam – problem focused

D0220 intraoral – periapical first radiographic image

Visit #2 (root canal began, but not completed)

D3999 unspecified endodontic procedure, by report

Visit #3 (root canal completed and core buildup placed)

D3330 endodontic therapy, molar (excluding final restoration)

D2950 core buildup, including any pins when required

Notes:

- No additional radiographs were billed after the preoperative, diagnostic radiograph
- The endodontic technologies that are used during the appointment are treated as a part of the root canal procedure itself.

CODING SCENARIO #2

Pulpectomy

A patient of record phones into your office and reports a severe toothache. The person did not sleep well last night and really needs to be seen by a dentist today. There is no room for them in your schedule, but you decide to work through lunch to see them.

They present to the office and a periapical radiograph is made. You perform a problem-focused exam and determine that they have irreversible pulpitis in the pulp of tooth #30. There is no time like the present – definitive treatment needs to be done so that they can begin to heal. Anesthetic was delivered to allow for a pulpal debridement to be done during this lunch break.

A complete pulpectomy was performed and a temporary restoration placed. Three weeks later, the patient returns for completion of the root canal and placement of a composite core restoration.

What procedure codes would be used to document and report the services provided during each of the two encounters?

Visit #1

D0140 limited exam – problem focused

D0220 intraoral – periapical first radiographic image

D3221 pulpal debridement, primary and permanent teeth

Visit #2

D3330 endodontic therapy, molar (excluding final restoration)

D2391 resin-based composite – one surface, posterior

Note: D2391 is the procedure is often used when there is a relatively uncomplicated restoration placed an access opening in a crown. For a more complicated restoration of an access hole a core buildup (D2950) and a new crown (e.g., D2740), procedures are likely to be delivered and reported.

CODING SCENARIO #3

Patient Referral for Apicoectomy

A patient presents to your office, referred by a friend who is a general dentist. The general dentist referred this patient for an "apico" for this person since she prefers not to do this type of procedure in her practice. You determine that both a periapical radiograph and a cone beam scan are needed to evaluate the complex case prior to determining the treatment plan.

This scan is evaluated and using the information found in the exam, the plane radiograph (PAX) and the CBCT, you determine that the apical surgery is the correct, best advice for treatment. (Remember to interpret the entire scan and to have a radiologist examine that scan as needed.) Included in the plan is a bone graft, which will be used due to the present of a large lesion that appears to have eroded both the buccal and palatal cortical plates of bone. A treatment plan is drawn up, consent is received and an appointment is made.

Note: A surgery of this nature is not often done on an emergency basis and often, an exam will be done on a day prior to the procedure.

The surgery is performed for tooth #3, on both the MB and DB roots. Both were resected, both received root-end fillings and when all was completed, a radiograph taken. Then, non-autogenous bone graft material was placed. There was no sinus perforation in the surgical field and it was determined that no barrier would be needed in this situation.

Sutures were placed and post-operative instructions given for a second time. The patient healed well during the first few days and was seen for suture removal. This appointment was uneventful and sutures were removed.

What procedure codes would be used to document and report the services provided during each of the three encounters?

Visit #1 (patient presents for diagnosis)

D0140 limited oral evaluation – problem focused

D0220 intraoral – periapical first radiographic image

and sometimes

D0230 intraoral – periapical – each additional radiographic image

Note: These images are often taken days prior to the procedure.

D0364 cone beam CT capture and interpretation with limited field of view – less than one whole jaw

Visit #2 (endodontic procedures delivered)

D3425 apicoectomy – molar (first root)

D3426 apicoectomy (each additional root)

D3430 retrograde filling – per root

D3430 retrograde filling – per root

Note: Root-end fillings are coded out per root. For a tooth #3, often there are two roots, which is why D3430 is reported twice.

D3428 bone graft in conjunction with periradicular surgery – per tooth single site

D3431 biologic materials to aid in soft and osseous tissue regeneration in conjunction with periradicular surgery

Visit #3 (post-operative follow-up)

D3999 unspecified endodontic procedure, by report

Note: Visit #3 is the suture removal appointment. It is considered part of the surgical care of the patient and no additional billing should be done.

CODING SCENARIO #4

Emergency Root Canal Patient

An emergency patient comes in and the dentist determines that she needs to start a root canal. The patient is in pain, but it's a case that fits easily into the dentist's typical endodontic abilities.

Let's say you are doing this for a patient of record at your dental office. The following codes would be utilized for what would be a typical and straight forward procedure, say for tooth #9:

D0140 limited oral evaluation – problem focused

D0220 intraoral – periapical first radiographic image

D3310 endodontic therapy, anterior tooth (excluding final restoration)

D2331 resin-based composite – two surfaces, anterior

What if I see them for a root canal appointment on emergency basis, then have to refer it out to a specialist?

In this case, where a general dentist opens a tooth on an emergency basis due to pain, and then feels the need to refer the case, the following codes could be utilized to document the situation:

D0140 limited oral evaluation – problem focused

D0220 intraoral – periapical first radiographic image

and sometimes

D0230 intraoral – periapical each additional radiographic image

D3221 pulp debridement, primary and permanent teeth

Notes: The pulpectomy (D3221) is done to alleviate acute pain. Temporary restorations are considered as a part of endodontic procedures.

A referral is then made to a new dentist. The new dentist would then also need to code a limited exam, make a new diagnostic preoperative radiograph to establish the new condition, and then perform the root canal and code for that. Next, the patient would need to have the permanent restoration done, a procedure which would depend on the existing restorative situation of the tooth.

CODING SCENARIO #5

Pulpal Regeneration

Visit #1

A 12-year-old patient presents with a parent to your clinic. Tooth #29 is somewhat painful, and the parent noticed that the child avoids chewing on the tooth.

After testing, the dentist can see and palpate mild swelling in the vestibule, buccal to the tooth. The tooth has never been restored. No caries is found on tooth #29, radiographically or clinically. It is percussion sensitive, palpation sensitive, slightly mobile (class I) and there are no probing depths over 3 mm. The tooth is sensitive to biting on the Tooth Slooth® and is not responsive to cold testing. Radiographically, one can see a moderately-sized PARL present around its apex. One can also visualize a very tall pulp chamber, even making the enamel look like a thin shell, rather than a thick band. The apex of the tooth has an immature foramen with no apical constriction and the apical opening being well over 1 mm wide. It appears that the tooth is 3-5 mm short of the length that it would normally achieve if the pulp had remained vital.

A diagnosis of pulp necrosis and acute apical abscess is made. The etiology is determined to be that a dens evaginatus tubercle must have broken off some time ago and led to the pulp necrosis. A treatment plan is discussed and with the parent's consent, it is decided to do a pulpal regeneration.

There is time in your schedule today and you have the training to know what treatment to do for the child. An access opening is made, the canal is appropriately instrumented and irrigated according to protocols established. An antibiotic paste is left in the canal system and a temporary restoration is placed.

What CDT Codes are applicable for the procedures delivered during this visit?

D0140 limited oral evaluation – problem focused

D0220 intraoral – periapical first radiographic image

D3355 pulpal regeneration – initial visit

Visit #2

The patient is asymptomatic at the second visit, three weeks after the first day you met. There is no swelling, the tooth is not abnormally mobile, and they can still not chew normally upon #29. It is decided that the case should be re-instrumented, re-irrigated and re-medicated. That is completed on this visit and a temporary restoration is replaced.

The CDT code for the second visit is:

D3356 pulpal regeneration – interim medication replacement

Visit #3

Three weeks have passed since the second visit. The tooth is now completely normal; all symptoms are gone. You decide to complete the case at this time. Anesthetic is given again, a dental dam placed again, and the canal space is re-irrigated to remove all the paste. Then a bioceramic plug is placed. It is delicately placed and tamped. After the apical barrier is stabilized, the canal is backfilled with gutta-percha. After that, a permanent, composite restoration is bonded in place. A final radiograph is made to demonstrate the result, to use as a baseline for future follow up. Annual follow ups will be conducted to monitor tooth #29. As its length increases, the dentin wall thickness increases. The apex will eventually "close" or become mature.

The CDT codes for this third visit are:

D3357 pulpal regeneration – completion of treatment

D2391 resin-based composite – one surface, posterior

CODING SCENARIO #6

Apicoectomy with Bony Defect

Day #1

Day #1 – A 36-year-old patient presented complaining of pain. Tooth #9 was very dark and non-vital gingiva was swollen and purulent. Radiographs show a huge PA area around #9. The patient stated that he had an accident on that tooth when he was a child. An antibiotic was prescribed.

Day #2 – The next morning the patient returned and the dentist performed root canal on #9 and was scheduled to return again that afternoon. In the afternoon the dentist opened a flap above #9 with the incision extending from distal of #8 to distal of #10. The flap revealed that buccal plate of bone around the apices was gone, and the whole area was a huge abscess and scar tissue. While curetting the bony defect, the dentist realized it went to the palatal plate of bone. At that point, the dentist did an apicoectomy on #9, irrigated the bony defect, and placed 2 gm of bone graft to preserve the bone and teeth #8 and 9.

How would these procedures be documented?

Day #1

Radiographs

D0220 intraoral – periapical first radiographic image

D0230 intraoral – periapical each additional radiographic image

Oral Evaluation

D0140 limited oral evaluation – problem focused

Prescribe antibiotic – No CDT Code

Note: D9630 is not applicable since its nomenclature states the procedure applies to drugs or medicaments dispensed in the office for home use, and its descriptor specifically excludes writing prescriptions.

Day #2 – Morning

Root canal on #9

D3310 endodontic therapy, anterior tooth (excluding final restoration)

Day #2 – Afternoon

Apicoectomy on #9

D3410 apicoectomy – anterior

Curetting the bony defect – No CDT Code; would be considered a component of D3410

Irrigated the bony defect – No CDT Code; would be considered a component of the graft procedure delivered at the same time

Placed 2 gm of bone graft to preserve the bone and teeth #8 and 9

D3428 bone graft in conjunction with periradicular surgery – per tooth, single site (and **D3429… each additional contiguous tooth in the same surgical site**, as the narrative indicates the graft affected two teeth)

Note: D7955 repair of maxillofacial soft and/or hard tissue defect could apply depending on how much the defect extended beyond the treated tooth, BUT this should not be reported in addition to D3428 or D3429.

CODING SCENARIO #7

Non-Carious Cervical Resorption Lesion

A patient presents with a tooth #18 that has a small invasive cervical resorption lesion on the buccal side. It was discovered during a routine hygiene appointment on a day when they were due for a set of BWX. The tooth has no pulpal symptoms, and no periapical symptoms. The lesion would probably be interpreted as caries by some dentists, but it is clear that there is no caries, as you cannot feel a cavitated lesion with any type of explorer. There is no periapical radiolucency.

The most definitive way to determine what to do with a resorption lesion that is diagnosed on regular plane radiography is to take a CBCT, small volume. This will help determine the exact location and size of the lesion. This helps determine if the lesion can be restored, should be left alone, or if the tooth is now unfixable or not restorable.

The CBCT scan is made and it is determined to be a Heithersay Class I or II lesion on the buccal surface of the tooth right at the height of the bony crest. It is determined that a flap procedure can be done to access this lesion which cannot be felt with a periodontal probe or any other explorer. The treatment plan is made to reflect a flap (D3427) and to periradicular surgery without apicoectomy. This flap is obviously required to access the lesion that can then be removed and restored.

When the flap is reflected, the lesion is removed, the lesion is treated to help stop any recurrent or continued procession of the lesion. The pulp chamber was not involved in the preparation of the tooth. The tooth is restored with some type of resin (often a true glass ionomer cement). The flap is sutured. Follow up is done over time to monitor pulpal health, as some of these can end up with pulpitis, just as a tooth with any carious lesion that has to be restored. But it is complicated by the fact that sometimes a resorption lesion can recur where a carious lesion would not.

How would you code for this scenario?

D0140 limited oral evaluation – problem focused

D0220 intraoral – periapical first radiographic image

D0365 cone beam CT capture and interpretation with field of view of one full dental arch – mandible

D3427 periradicular surgery without apicoectomy

D2391 resin-based composite – one surface, posterior

NOTE: In the past, many people would code out a regular apicoectomy code for this process, but that is not truly what was done. This code, D3427, more accurately describes what was done. That does not mean that this code will be covered by a given patient's insurance policy, even when it is clear that it is the best treatment for them.

Coding Q&A

1. **I worked really hard on a tooth that had six root canals in it and it seems like I should be able to have a code that shows how hard it was to do this case.**

   CDT codes for documenting and reporting endodontic therapy procedures by tooth type or location (e.g., anterior; premolar; molar) were established with CDT-1, effective January 1, 1990. This change replaced dental procedure codes based on number of canals per tooth (2, 3 or 4), plus a separate code for "each additional canal" that is used when needed. The rationale was that the change reflects what is most often encountered in clinical situations.

2. **I want to use an expensive adjunct irrigant, instead of, or in addition to, the traditional sodium hypochlorite that is so common. What code can I use to reflect the additional expertise and expense that it takes to use a material like that?**

   Irrigation as well as other parts of endodontic therapy are considered a part of the procedure itself and included in the code set for the type of tooth for which the root canal is being done. Removing a part of a procedure to make it separate and different when it is generally considered part of the procedure itself is often called "unbundling." From the ethical perspective both intentional unbundling to increase reimbursement, and intentional bundling to decrease reimbursement, are considered inappropriate.

3. **How can I use the CDT Code to describe that I have done an endodontic therapy in two visits instead of one visit? It costs the dentist more to do it in two visits and I think that should be reflected.**

   This is a common inquiry made to the American Association of Endodontists that has multiple parts. One question is about how to document the two visits. The first visit, when the need for RCT is diagnosed and then started, may be recorded with D3999 for record-keeping purposes. Then, at the second appointment, the typical D3330 code is used to reflect the completion of the treatment.

   The second, implied question seems to be more about how to charge more for the procedure than the dentist's established full D3330 fee. There is not a simple answer as every dentist is responsible for determining their fee and when doing so must consider the legal and ethical ramifications of having different full fees for the same procedure. This consideration should include a review your participating provider contracts in effect and discussion with your legal counsel.

4. What is the difference between using the apexification codes and the pulpal regeneration codes?

The procedures are very different in their intentions.

Apexification is the traditional way that dentistry solved the problem of teeth that had open, or immature, apices and needed root canals. Long-term calcium hydroxide treatment was used until the body made a hard tissue bridge over the apex. Then gutta-percha could be safely condensed against that bridge, in a manner that prevented the obturation from sliding long, into the periapical tissues. Pulpal regeneration is a different way to solve the problem in some of these very same cases that used to be solved with apexification.

However, in the pulpal regeneration procedure, the dentist is not trying to make a hard tissue apical barrier. Instead, he or she is simply trying to completely disinfect the canal system and to keep the stem cells alive near the apex. If the canal is sufficiently clean, and the stem cells are viable, a bioceramic barrier can be placed to the level of where a blood clot can be formed. Cervical to that barrier, the tooth is obturated and restored as if it had had a root canal done. Over time, the tooth will lengthen, the dentin walls will thicken and the apex will mature, closing in with a constriction as normal.

Summary

To sum up, when using Endodontics codes, remember to be aware of the main mistakes people make. Keep these things in mind:

- Billing out a root canal that was never actually finished may be the number one problem. This makes record keeping and fact finding extremely difficult. If you bill out a root canal as finished, but then do not finish it, you must make arrangements and explanations with any insurance company who you billed, the patient, and any other dentist to whom you have referred the case in order to have it completed. Remember to communicate well, using the codes as your language. Use the codes to state exactly what you have done to keep everyone in the loop.
- A major misuse of the code set is the overuse of code **D3331 treatment of a canal obstruction; non-surgical access**. The code is meant to be used fairly rarely and in extremely difficult cases. In a very difficult, calcified case where the root is more than 50% calcified, the code D3331 can be used. Another example of when to use this code is when a file has separated while another dentist was working on the tooth and the case is referred to a new dentist, who is then able to remove it, given that it took expertise or equipment to remove. The majority of root canals submitted to insurance companies by specialists do not include the D3331 code.
- As in every category, be sure to use the "additional" code numbers correctly. These codes sometimes are not used appropriately. Some other misuses include coding for intra-operative or post-operative radiographs, codes for additional dental material-based or technology-based steps that are generally considered standard parts of the root canal procedure.

Contributor Biography

Dr. Kenneth Wiltbank, D.M.D. is a practicing endodontist who owns and works in two practices in northwest Oregon. He also teaches at Oregon Health Sciences University as a part-time instructor. He has been involved with the American Association of Endodontists (AAE) since 2007, specifically as a member of the Scientific Review Board (reviewing articles for the Journal of Endodontics). He is also a member of the AAE's Dental Benefits Committee and the Practice Affairs Committee where he specialized in the AAE's relationships with the CDT codes and insurance companies. He is a voting member of the American Dental Association's Code Maintenance Committee, where he represents the AAE.

Chapter 5.
D4000 – D4999 Periodontics

By Marie Schweinebraten, D.D.S.

Introduction

Periodontal treatment has seen many changes over the last decade. For example, different types of grafting material, both autogenous and non-autogenous, are more common. Dental implants many times are included in periodontal treatment planning. Bone regeneration has become more predictable with the availability of new products and techniques. Periodontal procedure coding has grown with these changes as has the knowledge base required to code correctly and obtain reimbursement for the treatment completed.

Periodontics has always been a unique category because it has included both non-surgical and surgical procedures. What complicates matters is that some of the codes are site specific while others are tooth, quadrant (four or more teeth), or area (one to three teeth) specific. Adding to the confusion is that procedure codes have become differentiated as to the type of material used as well as to whether the procedure is performed on a tooth or implant. There are also many periodontal codes that overlap with codes from other categories.

Coding for periodontal procedures also may require the use of "á la carte" codes. Bone graft materials, for example, are listed separately from the procedure for achieving access – osseous surgery (D4260 or D4261) or gingival flap (D4240 or D4241). There are also separate codes for other procedures that may be required in a graft case, including placement of barrier membranes or biologic materials to aid in regeneration. Thus, for a given outcome there could be a number of separate procedures involved, each documented with its individual CDT code.

It is especially important in the periodontal category to realize that procedure codes are meant to describe the treatment rendered, not the means that are used to accomplish the treatment. For example, a gingivectomy can be done by several techniques, including utilizing a blade, a periodontal knife or a laser. The code for the procedure, however, is the same.

With attention to detail and a basic understanding of periodontal treatment and the codes, a dental office can prevent confusion for the patient and misunderstanding of plan coverage while at the same time obtaining reimbursement as effectively and efficiently as possible.

Key Definitions and Concepts

Full quadrant: A section of the mouth with four or more contiguous teeth or tooth spaces.

Partial quadrant: A section of the mouth with one to three contiguous teeth or tooth spaces

Site: The term site is use to describe a single area, or position. "Site" is frequently used to describe an area of recession on a single tooth or an osseous defect adjacent to a single tooth. It can also apply to soft tissue or osseous defects in an edentulous area.

For example:

- If two contiguous teeth have areas of recession, each area is a single site.
- If two contiguous teeth have adjacent but separate osseous defects, each defect is a single site.
- If these defects communicate, however, they swould be considered a single site.
- In an edentulous area, up to two contiguous edentulous tooth positions may be considered a single site.

Tooth bounded space: a space created by one or more missing teeth that have a tooth on each side of the edentulous area.

Autogenous soft tissue graft: Graft material is taken from the patient's oral cavity. There is a second surgical site in the patient's mouth.

Non-autogenous: There is no second surgical site in the patient's mouth. The graft material comes from another source. An example is AlloDerm.

D4999 unspecified periodontal procedure, by report: This code may apply when a provider feels there is no specific code for the procedure completed. In these cases, a narrative or report is necessary to explain the unusual circumstance.

Changes to This Category

There are two changes in the periodontal category in CDT 2019. Both are revisions, and address anatomical crown exposure. The changes better define the use of four or more teeth or tooth bounded spaces per quadrant and one to three teeth or tooth bounded spaces per quadrant.

D4230 anatomical crown exposure-four or more contiguous teeth or tooth bounded ~~tooth~~ spaces per quadrant
This procedure is utilized in an otherwise periodontally healthy area to remove enlarged gingival tissue and supporting bone (ostectomy) to provide anatomically correct gingival relationship.

D4231 anatomical crown exposure-one to three teeth or tooth bounded ~~tooth~~ spaces per quadrant
This procedure is utilized in an otherwise periodontally healthy area to remove enlarged gingival tissue and supporting bone (ostectomy) to provide an anatomically correct gingival relationship.

The changes better define the area where the crown exposure is performed. For example, even though a tooth #10 may be missing, if anatomical crown lengthening is necessary on teeth #9 and #11, correct coding would be D4231 since treatment would involve the edentulous area. Elevation of the flap to treat teeth #9 and #11 would require some revision of the tissue where tooth #10. Thus, the correct description includes a tooth bounded space.

Diagnosis Codes – ICD-10-CM

The CDT to ICD tables in Appendix 1 provide appropriate guidance on linkages between Periodontics procedure codes and diagnosis codes. This chapter does not contain supplemental information on this topic.

CODING SCENARIO #1

Periodontal Abscess

A patient presented in pain and complaining about swelling around one tooth. The doctor's emergency evaluation focused on the patient's complaint and included two periapical radiographic images and pocket measurements of the teeth in the area. The swelling was clearly adjacent to tooth #3 and the sulcus gushed a purulent mixture of blood and pus when probed.

The doctor treated the patient for a periodontal abscess by debridement and draining through the sulcus, irrigating the pocket with chlorhexidine and prescribing the patient an antibiotic.

How could this encounter be coded?

Since the evaluation was both problem-focused and limited to the patient's complaint, the appropriate codes for diagnostic procedures would be:

D0140 limited oral evaluation – problem focused

D0220 intraoral – periapical first radiographic image

D0230 intraoral – periapical each additional radiographic image

In this case there are a number of codes that might be used to document the operative services, alone or in combination. Possible procedure coding options are:

D9110 palliative (emergency) treatment of dental pain – minor procedure

Use of this code to document the service provided may require a narrative to describe the exact treatment rendered. It may be the most appropriate code to use in this case. The following code may also be considered:

D7510 incision and drainage of abscess – intraoral soft tissue

CODING SCENARIO #2

Chronic Generalized Periodontitis

A 49-year-old male patient presents for periodontal examination with a chief complaint of sore and bleeding gums. Medical history is significant for type II diabetes being treated with Metformin (glucophage), and hypertension which was being treated with a calcium channel blocker (nifedipine-adalat). His last dental appointment was five years ago and there are heavy accumulations of plaque and calculus, both supra-gingival and sub-gingival.

Since the amount of calculus and plaque prevented a periodontal evaluation from being performed adequately, the patient was seen by the hygienist that same day. Without using any anesthesia, she utilized an ultrasonic scaler to debride supragingival calculus and plaque in all four quadrants. After reviewing home care instructions and giving the patient chlorhexidine rinse, provided by the office, the patient was scheduled to return in two weeks for a periodontal evaluation and appropriate radiographic images.

How would these visits be coded?

Initial Visit: Assessment and Debridement

D0191 assessment of a patient

D4355 full mouth debridement to enable comprehensive oral evaluation and diagnosis on a subsequent visit

D1330 oral hygiene instructions

D9630 drugs or medicaments dispensed in the office for home use

Second Visit: Evaluation, Diagnosis and Treatment Planning

Two weeks later, the patient returned for radiographic images and a complete periodontal evaluation.

The diagnosis is chronic generalized periodontitis with pocket depths ranging from 4 to 9 millimeters, furcation invasion, mobility, and localized recession. There are interproximal papillae that exhibit swelling with a "granulated" surface appearance to the soft tissue resembling hyperplasia possibly caused by a calcium channel-blocking drug. Consultation with the patient's internist to evaluate possibility of changing high blood pressure medication was done by the dentist.

A complete oral evaluation with panoramic and full mouth periapical radiographic images were taken. The diagnostic findings were:

1. Missing teeth #1, 5, 12, 16, 17, 21, 28 and 32. The premolars were extracted for orthodontic reasons when he was a teenager.
2. Bone loss of up to 40 percent around the posterior teeth with pocket depths ranging from 5 to 9 mm in the posterior.
3. Heavy accumulations of plaque and calculus supra and sub-gingival
4. Moderate generalized gingival overgrowth probably related to his calcium channel medication
5. Furcation involvement on the molars
6. Mobility of teeth
7. Inadequate oral hygiene

The evaluation and diagnosis led to a multiple appointment treatment plan for this patient – four quadrants of scaling and root planing spread across two appointments, and a third appointment four to six weeks after the SRP for a post-operative visit to assess the outcome.

CDT codes for the services delivered and planned during the second visit follow:

D0150 **comprehensive oral evaluation – new or established patient**

or **D0180** **comprehensive periodontal evaluation-new or established patient**

D0210 **intraoral – complete series of radiographic images**

D0330 **panoramic radiographic image**

D1330 **oral hygiene instructions**

D9311 **consultation with a medical health care professional**

Treatment Visit #1: SRP – two quadrants

D4341 periodontal scaling and root planning – four or more teeth per quadrant

Note: This procedure is reported twice and the two quadrants treated (e.g., maxillary right and mandibular right) are identified.

Treatment Visit #2: SRP – two quadrants

D4341 periodontal scaling and root planning – four or more teeth per quadrant

This procedure is reported twice and the two quadrants treated (e.g., maxillary left and mandibular left) are identified.

Post-Op Visit: 4-6 weeks after SRP completed

D0171 re-evaluation – post operative office visit

Post-scaling and root planing, re-charting was done at this appointment, noting that significant pocket depth with bleeding on probing in the posterior areas was evident. The dentist felt that the patient would benefit from osseous surgery in the posterior quadrants (D4260) at a later date. The medical consultation from the first appointment was returned and the physician plans to change the patient's hypertension medication.

CODING SCENARIO #3

Treatment to Eliminate Periodontal Pocketing

A 60-year-old female has been under care since having scaling and root planing done eight months ago, followed by periodic periodontal maintenance (D4910) every three months. The patient decided she is ready to proceed with planned treatment to eliminate periodontal pocketing, but is very anxious about the surgery. Before proceeding, the doctor completed a new periodontal chart to assess her current situation. Since the full mouth radiographs were less than a year old, no additional radiographs were necessary.

The diagnostic findings are as follows:

1. Missing teeth #1, 2, 16, 17, 18, and 32
2. Bone loss is generalized and ranges from 10-50 percent with periodontal pocket depths up to 5 to 9 mm
3. Furcation involvement in the molar areas
4. Vertical defects on the distal of tooth #19 and the mesial of tooth #21
5. Tooth mobility
6. Periodontal bleeding on probing in the periodontal pocket areas
7. Patient apprehension to dental treatment

What CDT code is used to report the periodontal charting completed at this appointment?

Charting is considered to be a part of a comprehensive periodontal evaluation (**D0180**), which also should include details such as bleeding on probing, furcation involvement, mobility, recession, and clinical attachment loss. These findings may also be part of a comprehensive oral evaluation (**D0150**). It is recommended that periodontal charting and evaluation be completed annually for patients with a history of periodontitis.

The patient's next appointment was for four quadrants of osseous surgery and bone grafts to address the defects on teeth #19 and 21. These procedures would be delivered with the patient under conscious sedation due to her anxiety.

Services delivered during this appointment would be coded as follows:

For four quadrants of osseous surgery:

D4260 osseous surgery (includes elevation of a full thickness flap and closure) – four of more contiguous teeth or tooth bounded spaces per quadrant

Note: This procedure is reported four times as it is a "per quadrant" service and all four quadrants were involved (maxillary right and left; mandibular right and left) on this date of service.

For tooth #19 (distal):

D4263 **bone replacement graft-retained natural tooth first site in quadrant**

and **D4265** **biologic material to aid in osseous tissue regeneration**

For tooth #21 (mesial):

D4264 **bone replacement graft-retained natural tooth each additional site in quadrant**

and **D4265** **biologic material to aid in osseous regeneration**

For 2.5 hours of anesthesia:

D9239 **intravenous moderate (conscious) sedation/analgesia – first 15 minutes**

D9243 **intravenous moderate (conscious) sedation – each subsequent 15 minute increment**

Note: Since the anesthesia procedure took 2.5 hours (150 minutes) and these codes are reported in 15-minute increments, the patient record and claim would document the first 15 minutes of sedation, D9239, once and then document the additional 135 minutes with D9243 and a "Quantity" of nine.

The patient returned for a post-surgery check two weeks later for suture removal, light cleansing of the affected areas, and oral hygiene instructions. At that time, the doctor determined that the patient would benefit from an antimicrobial mouth rinse (chlorhexidine), which the office provided.

CDT Codes for this visit are:

D9430 **office visit for observation (during regularly scheduled hours) – no other services performed**

D9630 **drugs or medicaments dispensed in the office for home use**

CODING SCENARIO #4

Orthodontic Patient with Gingival Inflammation

A patient, who is a teenager in active orthodontic treatment, comes in for a prophylaxis every three to four months. She struggles with homecare and, as a result, the gingiva is bleeding and tender with enlarged tissue, actually covering some of the brackets. Her medical history is within normal limits. There is no bone loss as determined by a panoramic radiograph taken six months ago. In addition, scaling is difficult with brackets and appliances present. This is a three-appointment scenario.

How would the appointments be coded?

Visit #1

An examination was done with periodontal charting that included notation of bleeding points and pocketing. Homecare instructions were reinforced, and all tissues were irrigated with chlorhexidine rinse. Extra-oral photographs were taken to document the hyperplastic tissue. The patient was scheduled for a gingivectomy in four full quadrants.

CDT codes for the first appointment's procedures are:

D0180 comprehensive periodontal evaluation, new or established patient

D0350 2D facial photographic image obtained intra-orally or extra-orally

D1330 oral hygiene instructions

D4921 gingival irrigation – per quadrant

Note: D4921 is reported four times as all quadrants of the mouth received gingival irrigation.

Visit #2

The patient received a gingivectomy in each quadrant. These procedures were completed using local anesthesia for patient comfort and with a laser for the instrumentation.

CDT codes for the second appointment's procedures are:

D4210 gingivectomy or gingivoplasty – four or more contiguous teeth or tooth bounded spaces per quadrant

Note: D4210 should be reported with a quantity of four as all quadrants of the mouth received gingivectomy. Use of a laser in this procedure is not relevant from the coding perspective as the code documents the treatment done, not the specific instrument or technique used to perform the gingivectomy.

Although there is a statement at the beginning of the Periodontics category of service indicating that local anesthesia is usually considered to be part of periodontal procedures, this does not preclude documenting and reporting its delivery with the following CDT code:

D9215 local anesthesia in conjunction with operative or surgical procedures

Visit #3

The patient was seen a month later for follow-up, with no services provided, and the CDT code for this encounter is:

D0171 re-evaluation – post-operative visit

The patient should then be placed on a periodontal maintenance schedule since active periodontal treatment was rendered. It is important to remember, however, that carriers have plan limitations, which may reimburse only a limited number of prophylaxes or periodontal maintenance visits per year. This may also apply to comprehensive examinations. In unusual cases, a narrative may explain the need for additional treatment outside the plan limitation.

CODING SCENARIO #5

Scaling in the Presence of Mucositis Around an Implant

A patient of record who has been on periodic maintenance visits (D4910) presents for this visit with the complaint of soreness around the implant for tooth #5. Examination revealed bleeding with probing around the implant accompanied by with swelling and some suppuration. Resulting pocket depths were 4-5mm. A periapical radiograph was taken, which indicated bone height comparable to that seen previously.

The doctor treated this area with debridement and curettage of the area through the gingival sulcus. The periodic maintenance visit is not done at this appointment.

How would this encounter be coded?

Visit #1

D0140 limited oral evaluation – problem focused

D0220 intra oral – periapical radiograph radiographic image

D6081 scaling and debridement in the presence of inflammation or mucositis of a single implant, including cleaning of the implant surfaces, without flap entry and closure

The D6081 procedure is not performed in conjunction with D1110, D4910, or D4346.

Subsequent Visits

Continuation of periodic periodontal maintenance plan, each reported with:

D4910 periodontal maintenance

CODING SCENARIO #6

Ailing Failing Implant

Visit #1

The patient presents with the chief complaint of soreness and bleeding associated with a restored implant #19. Evaluation of the area reveals a 7 mm pocketing surrounding the implant with bleeding on probing. No mobility in the implant is detected. A periapical radiographic image reveals circumferential bone loss approaching the middle level of the bone on the implant, an increase from previous radiographs. It was determined that the implant was treatable. The patient was placed on an appropriate antibiotic and scheduled to return for treatment.

How would this encounter be coded?

D0140 limited oral evaluation – problem focused

D0220 intraoral – periapical first radiograph image

Visit #2

The patient returned in 10 days and the swelling had subsided. Under oral sedation and local anesthesia, full thickness mucoperiosteal flaps were elevated and the implant surface was debrided with saline, scaled with an ultrasonic implant tip, and then treated with chlorhexidine solution. The site was grafted with bone and covered with a resorbable barrier and closed with sutures.

How would this encounter be coded?

This encounter would be coded as:

D9248 non-intravenous conscious sedation

D6101 debridement of a peri-implant defect or defects surrounding a single implant, and surface cleaning of the exposed implant surfaces, including flap entry and closure.

D4921 gingival irrigation-per quadrant

D6103 bone graft for repair of peri-implant defect-does not include flap entry and closure

D4266 guided tissue regeneration – resorbable barrier, per site

CODING SCENARIO #7

Overdue Patient with Gingivitis

A patient of record in the office has not been seen for over two years. When they arrive for a routine prophylaxis, the evaluation reveals heavy plaque, some supra- and sub-gingival calculus, with moderate stain. Bleeding on probing is noted on most teeth accompanied by edema and swelling. No bone loss is seen on bitewing radiographs that are taken. From the clinical evaluation, a diagnosis of generalized moderate to severe gingivitis is made. The hygienist proceeds with a full mouth scaling treatment, not a prophylaxis, noting that this scaling procedure requires more time than needed for a prophylaxis.

How should this appointment be coded for reimbursement?

Since the patient has not been seen in the office for over a year, a comprehensive evaluation should be done. This includes both dental and periodontal charting, with pocket depths, bleeding points, and any additional findings such as suppuration and edema.

D0150 comprehensive oral evaluation-new or established patient

or **D0180 comprehensive periodontal evaluation-new or established patient**

As mentioned, bitewing radiographs were also taken.

D0274 bitewings – four radiographic images

It is recommended that patients have a panoramic radiograph or full mouth radiographs every five years. If this patient does not have either in the last five years, then most likely a panoramic radiograph would also be taken.

D0330 panoramic radiographic image

In this case, a comprehensive oral evaluation has been done and treatment will be done at the same visit. Since the diagnosis is generalized moderate to severe gingivitis, treatment will be more difficult and require more time than a routine adult prophylaxis.

D4346 scaling in the presence of generalized moderate or severe gingival inflammation-full mouth, after oral evaluation

This scenario emphasizes that an evaluation can be done the same day as treatment when scaling is coded as D4346. The D4346 procedure differs from **D4355 full mouth debridement to enable a comprehensive oral evaluation and a diagnosis on a subsequent visit** as this procedure addresses removal of accumulations and inflammation present that do not allow a comprehensive evaluation to be done. For example, pocket depths cannot be recorded due to the amount of calculus present both supra- and sub-gingivally. These cases require a healing period to accurately do the evaluation and make a diagnosis.

Also note that D4346 is a full mouth procedure. It cannot be coded multiple times by quadrant.

Many times a second procedure of scaling may be necessary to accomplish adequate debridement for patients who have had the D4346 procedure. For example, a re-evaluation (**D0171 re-evaluation-post-operative office visit**) might be appropriate, or a second appointment for a prophylaxis (**D1110**) if inflammation and pocket depths have decreased.

As with all codes, carriers differ as to the benefit allowed for D4346. A clinician should code for what they do, not code for reimbursement. Also remember that unless a new code is used appropriately and submitted, carriers will not have a history of the frequency of use or the dentist's full fee for the procedure.

CODING SCENARIO #8

Foreign Object Stuck Between Teeth

A patient comes in for an emergency visit. Something is "stuck" between teeth #19 and 20 and is causing some swelling and pain. The patient has not been able brush or floss the area and resolve the issue. After examining the area and taking a periapical radiograph, you decide the problem has not caused any bone loss or is endodontically related. Infiltrating the interproximal area and scaling, you find a husk from popcorn, which is removed. After giving post-operative instructions, the patient is dismissed.

How should this be coded?

In this case, the exam should be coded:

D0140 limited oral evaluation – problem focused

A periapical radiograph was taken.

D0220 intraoral – periapical first radiographic image

Treatment the swelling and pain can be coded in various ways depending on what procedures have been delivered, using a code's nomenclature and descriptor as the guide. D9110 would be the most likely one to describe the service provided. It can be used in conjunction with D9215 local anesthesia in conjunction with operative or surgical procedures. At times, carriers request a narrative to explain the rationale for the procedure.

D9110 palliative (emergency) treatment of dental pain – minor procedure
This is typically reported on a "per visit" basis for emergency treatment of dental pain.

In cases where D7510 is appropriate, the lesion will not only exhibit swelling and bleeding on probing, but will also have suppuration or exudate when scaled. This occurs frequently when periodontal pockets are present.

D7510 Incision and drainage of abscess-intraoral soft tissue Involves incision through mucosa, including periodontal origins

An alternative is **D4999 unspecified periodontal procedure, by report**, if the clinician feels that the lesion may result in periodontal complications or signs and symptoms found are primarily periodontal. Again, a narrative would be necessary to describe the treatment provided when submitted for reimbursement. Many carriers do not reimburse "999" codes. But always remember, you should code for what you do.

CODING SCENARIO #9

Scaling and Root Planing of Only Three Quadrants

A patient presents at the office and requires three posterior quadrants of scaling and root planing. The fourth quadrant has no periodontal disease, but does require a prophylaxis. All treatment is completed after two appointments.

Visit #1: Evaluation, Diagnosis and Treatment Planning

We assume that this patient has been seen for an evaluation, perhaps at the time they were scheduled for a prophylaxis. If so it would be correct to code for an evaluation and the adult prophylaxis.

D0150 comprehensive oral evaluation – new or established patient

or **D0180 comprehensive periodontal evaluation – new or established patient**

D1110 prophylaxis – adult

Note that this will be a comprehensive evaluation since it has been determined that the patient requires periodontal therapy. Periodontal charting including pocket depths and current radiographs will be necessary to support the need for scaling and root planing.

Visit #2: SRP – Three Quadrants

At a subsequent appointment, the scaling and root planing can be performed. In some instances, performing a prophylaxis prior to scaling and root planing can decrease the inflammation and allow a more thorough debridement during scaling and root planing since bleeding will be less and access to subgingival calculus and toxins is improved.

Note: It is always advisable to request a pre-treatment estimate prior to any periodontal therapy since carriers may have plan limitations that may affect reimbursement. For example, some carriers will only reimburse a maximum of two quadrants of scaling and root planing per appointment.

The bottom line is that you could submit for three quadrants of scaling and root planing and a "prophylaxis" for the fourth quadrant, but in most instances it would not be reimbursed in full.

D4342 periodontal scaling and root planing – one to three teeth per quadrant

Note: D4342 is reported three times and the three quadrants treated are identified.

1. **Our patient has pocketing and an osseous defect on the distal of the last tooth in a quadrant. All other teeth in the quadrant have pockets that are three millimeters or less. We are not sure whether the treatment procedure to report is osseous surgery (D4261) or a distal wedge (D4274). Which is appropriate?**

   If there is an osseous defect evident radiographically on the distal of the last tooth in a quadrant, and treatment of the defect includes osseous contouring and possibly a bone graft, then the treatment should be coded as osseous surgery one to three teeth, D4261. If a bone graft is used, use D4263 or appropriate codes for membranes or biologics if they, too, apply.

   If the procedure involves only removal of soft tissue and debridement of the tooth surface, then the mesial/distal wedge procedure would apply. According to D4274, the descriptor states that "This procedure is performed in an edentulous area adjacent to a tooth, allowing removal of a tissue wedge to gain access for debridement, permit close flap adaptation, and reduce pocket depths." No osseous contouring or regeneration is done, but a flap is elevated and the area debrided including scaling and root planing.

2. **What is the code for reporting platelet rich plasma (PRP)?**

   Platelet rich plasma (PRP) is a concentrated suspension of the growth factors found in platelets. It is a procedure where a patient's blood is drawn and then centrifuged to obtain the PRP. This procedure should be coded using **D7921 collection and application of autogenous blood concentrate product**.

3. **We use the bone replacement graft codes D4263 and D4264 for periodontal defects around and adjacent to natural teeth. Do we use the same codes in periodontal defects around existing implants?**

   There are distinct codes for bone grafts around natural teeth and those around implants. If natural teeth are being treated, then D4263 and D4264 should be submitted. These codes apply "per site." If a bone graft is placed around an existing implant, then **D6103 bone graft for repair of peri-implant defect – does not include flap entry and closure** would be correct.

4. **We use the bone replacement graft code D7953 when placing graft material in an extraction socket when removing a natural tooth. But if we place an immediate implant in the extraction site and place a bone graft around the implant, do we still use D7953 or do we use one of the periodontal bone graft codes D4263 or D4264?**

   The nomenclature for D7953 indicates that this procedure is appropriate to report when the service is for ridge preservation, and the code's descriptor also makes reference to "preservation of ridge integrity...clinically indicated in preparation for implant reconstruction." D4263 and D4264 specifically state that they apply to "natural" teeth. The only appropriate code to use which would apply when placing an immediate implant and simultaneously placing bone graft material around the implant would be **D6104 bone graft at time of implant placement**. Note that the descriptor states that if a barrier membrane or biologic materials are used to aid in osseous regeneration, these should be reported separately using the D4265, D4266 or D4267.

5. **If we remove an existing implant, and place a bone graft in the site, can we use the D7953 code?**

   Yes. You should be using two codes to describe what you are doing. The first would be D6100 Implant removal, by report and the second should be D7953 which states that the graft "is placed in an extraction or implant removal site at the time of extraction or removal." This descriptor statement means D7953 is appropriate in this situation.

6. **The dental hygienists in our office are using Oraqix prior to scaling and root planing. How would Oraqix be reported?**

   The periodontics category of service indicates that "Local anesthesia is usually considered to be part of periodontal procedures." As Oraqix is a topical local anesthetic its application would be recorded as **D9215 local anesthesia in conjunction with operative or surgical procedures**.

7. **What code should I use to report periodontal charting?**

   There is no separate code for periodontal charting. It is considered to be part of a comprehensive periodontal evaluation (D0180) or may be part of a comprehensive oral evaluation (D0150). It could also be considered part of a re-evaluation, such as that done after initial therapy.

8. **Does D4910 periodontal maintenance include an evaluation?**

   The procedure does not include an evaluation. If one is performed, the type of diagnostic evaluation should be reported separately. In most cases, **D0120 periodic oral evaluation-established patient**. If a more comprehensive evaluation is done then **D0150 comprehensive oral evaluation, new or established patient** or **D0180 comprehensive periodontal evaluation-new or established patient** would be appropriate.

9. **A patient needs multiple connective tissue grafts in the mandible. There are three to six millimeters of recession on the facial of teeth #23, 24, 25, 26, 27, and 28, with no attached gingiva. There is also no attached gingiva around the implant in the area of #29. The dentist plans on using Alloderm when performing connective tissue grafts on all involved teeth and the implant during one appointment.**

   Should I just submit a code for the first tooth and then one code for the remaining teeth since they are contiguous? How do we submit for a soft tissue graft around an implant? And which connective graft code would apply, D4273 or D4275?

   In this case, the appropriate code would be **D4275 non-autogenous connective tissue graft procedure** for the first tooth involved. You would then use **D4285** for grafts to each of the additional teeth or implants involved. In this specific case, D4275 would be submitted one time and D4285 would be submitted six times.

10. **I have many orthodontic patients who come in for a prophylaxis. Sometimes we find the tissue around brackets and wires is hyperplastic and bleeding with generalized pseudo-pocketing. There is no bone loss evident and homecare is poor. Although the hygienist spends more time on these patients than she would with a routine prophylaxis patient, we still have to code it as a D1110. Is this the only option for coding that we have?**

    The code for scaling in the presence of moderate to severe inflammation (D4346) would be appropriate in this case. Scaling and root planing is not necessary but the procedure is more involved than a routine prophylaxis. It does include full mouth. And remember that carriers may vary on the documentation required when submitting for reimbursement and limitations on the number of times this procedure is covered.

11. **My patient has had periodontal treatment in the past and is on periodic periodontal maintenance (D4910). The patient changed dental insurance and when we filed for our visit, the coverage was denied due to no history of periodontal treatment. What would best resolve this issue?**

    You should send in the current periodontal charting, radiographs and the patient's history of prior periodontal treatment. Ask for a review of the claim. Some insurers require periodontal treatment in the prior 24 months to be eligible.

12. **I plan anatomic crown exposure on teeth #27, 29, and 30. #28 is missing but this area will be involved in the procedure to achieve anatomically correct gingival relationships. Should I code this as D4230 or D4231?**

    As four or more teeth or tooth bounded spaces (#28) are involved, you would code this as **D4230**. A tooth bounded space is a space created by one or more missing teeth that has a tooth on each side.

13. **I have a new patient that has so much plaque and calculus that it is difficult to determine a treatment plan. After doing a full mouth debridement and now being able to determine the patient's dental problems, can I do the exam on the same day?**

    No. The CDT 2018 revision to **D4355 full mouth debridement to enable a comprehensive oral evaluation and diagnosis on a subsequent visit** makes it clear that the exam must be done on a separate day. This allows healing of the inflamed tissues and results in the ability to perform an evaluation.

14. **A periodontal maintenance patient presents with a localized area of pocketing with 6 mm probing depths. If I treat this area today, is this included in the D4910 periodontal maintenance, whose descriptor indicates site specific scaling and root planing? Or can it be coded as D4342 scaling and root planing – one to three teeth per quadrant?**

    The descriptor of D4910 includes site specific scaling and root planing. It is considered part of the periodontal maintenance appointment on the same day. If the change is significant, you may want to obtain a current periodontal chart and a radiographic image for the patient and then consider scaling and root planing (D4342) with local anesthesia as a separate procedure. It is advantageous to have periodontal charting that demonstrates an increase in pocket depths that support the need for scaling and root planing.

Summary

Filing for benefits related to periodontal procedures can be frustrating. In order to reduce issues with carriers and patients, some things can be routinely be done to avoid problems. Use this checklist as a reminder:

- Obtain proper documentation when evaluating a patient who requires periodontal treatment. A full periodontal charting should be present, which includes not only pocket depths, but also recession, amount of attached gingiva, furcation involvement, mobility, bleeding on probing, clinical attachment loss and any other periodontal condition found. The charting should be recent, usually less than six months old. Radiographic images should typically be less than one year old. Periapical images are preferred over bitewing or panoramic images. At times, especially for soft tissue grafts, photographic images may be helpful, but these are not normally submitted with the initial claim
- A pre-treatment estimate is the best way to avoid problems with reimbursement. Although not a guarantee of benefits, it establishes guidelines for the patient related to payments. With some plans, pre-treatment estimates may be valid for a limited time and this should be taken into consideration.
- When submitting for periodontal reimbursement, attachments are essential. For scaling and root planing, as well as osseous surgery, periapical radiographs and charting are necessary. For soft tissue grafting, recession and the amount of attached gingiva must be evident on the charting. If initial therapy has been performed prior to any necessary osseous surgery, many carriers will require periodontal charting after the scaling and root planing has healed and prior to the osseous surgery for comparison pocket depths. This holds true for periodontal maintenance patients also. If it is determined that treatment such as scaling and root planing or osseous surgery is needed and a patient has been on a periodontal maintenance schedule, then previous, as well as recent charting, should be available to demonstrate changes, normally seen as increased pocket depths between appointments.

Contributor Biography

Marie Schweinebraten, D.M.D. is a practicing periodontist in Duluth, GA. She has been active in the dental tripartite, including serving on the ADA Council on Dental Benefit Programs and as Fifth District Trustee. She participated as an ADA representative on the Code Revision and Maintenance Committees for seven years. Presently she serves as Insurance Consultant for the American Academy of Periodontology, representing the AAP on the Code Maintenance Committee the past five years. Dr. Schweinebraten has given code workshops and is a certified insurance consultant.

Chapter 6. D5000 – D5899 Prosthodontics, Removable

By Terry Kelly, D.M.D.

Introduction

The Removable Prosthodontics category of service describes procedures which replace missing dentition in partially or completely edentulous patients. Stability and retention of a removable prosthesis may be dependent on both hard and soft tissue support, which may also include dental implants. Many of the materials used in the fabrication of these prostheses have particular characteristics that are described in the code. These characteristics identify their uniqueness and create specific instances where they should be used.

In addition, because most of the materials used can be modified or repaired for an otherwise well-fitting prosthesis, there is a significant portion of this code set which describes various repairs, relines, and adjustments which can be incorporated to maintain or modify a prosthesis when changes occur to the supporting structures. It is important to note that all procedure codes in this category are inherently based on either a partial or complete denture. Moreover, most of the procedures will specifically designate maxillae or mandible in the nomenclature of the code.

Key Definitions and Concepts

The Glossary of Prosthodontics Terms from the Academy of Prosthodontics contains descriptors for all removable prosthodontic procedures, and is an excellent resource for comprehensive definitions of prosthodontic procedures. It is available at *www.academyofprosthodontics.org*.

Complete Denture: A removable prosthesis that replaces an entire arch of dentition and associated structures.

Partial Denture: A removable prosthesis that replaces a portion of missing dentition and associated structures.

Immediate Partial or Complete Denture: A removable prosthesis that is specifically designed to replace a portion or all of the missing dentition in an arch, which is inserted immediately following extraction of teeth. Adaptation of the prosthesis frequently involves placement of a soft lining material at insertion, which is included as part of the routine delivery of care for these procedure codes. Subsequent visits which may include additional adjustments or relines should be coded as such. It is important to note that an immediate denture is only applicable as a coded procedure for the initial insertion appointment. After that, for purposes of adjustments, repairs, or relines, the correct code would either be a partial or complete denture.

Overdenture: A removable prosthesis that covers and is partially supported by natural teeth, roots, and/or dental implants.

Prosthesis: An artificial replacement of an absent part of the human body; designed to restore form and function.

Changes to This Category

The codes describing resin based partial dentures now include "retentive/clasping materials" in the nomenclature to better describe the retentive element of the prosthesis. There are two new codes and four revised codes:

D5282 removable unilateral partial denture – one piece cast metal (including clasps and teeth), mandibular

D5283 removable unilateral partial denture – one piece cast metal (including clasps and teeth), maxillary

D5211 maxillary partial denture – resin base (including any conventional clasps retentive/clasping materials, rests, and teeth)
Includes acrylic resin base denture with resin or wrought wire clasps.

D5212 mandibular partial denture – resin base (including any conventional clasps retentive/clasping materials, rests, and teeth)
Includes acrylic resin base denture with resin or wrought wire clasps.

D5630 repair or replace broken clasp retentive/clasping materials – per tooth

This allows more accurate coding for materials other than a metal clasp when used for retention of a tooth – supported partial denture for existing codes D5211, D5212, and D5630.

Other changes include a new code to describe reinforcement of a complete denture with the addition of a metal substructure embedded in the denture base:

D5876 add metal sub structure to acrylic full denture (per arch)

One code has been deleted:

D5281 removable unilateral partial denture – one piece cast metal (including clasps and teeth)

Diagnosis Codes – ICD-10-CM

The CDT to ICD tables in Appendix 1 provide appropriate guidance on linkages between removable Prosthodontics procedure codes and diagnosis codes. This chapter does not contain supplemental information on this topic.

CODING SCENARIO #1

Modified Mandibular Complete Denture

A patient presents with an existing mandibular complete denture which needs to be modified following placement of two implant fixtures in the anterior mandible. Following surgery the denture is relieved in the areas of implant placement, and a soft liner or tissue conditioner is placed to re-adapt the denture base.

How would you code these procedures?

D5875 modification of removable prosthesis following implant surgery

D5851 tissue conditioning, mandible

Notes:

- **D5875** is used to describe the procedure which modifies an existing removable prosthesis following implant surgery.
- In the event that a completely new mandibular overdenture will be fabricated with an implant abutment/attachment such as a locator, then the following codes in the Implant Services category would apply:

D6111 implant/abutment supported removable denture for edentulous arch – mandible

D6052 semi-precision attachment abutment

(Report each abutment attachment assembly separately.)

CODING SCENARIO #2

Removable Partial Denture and Bone Loss

A patient presents with an existing mandibular removable partial denture which is supported by remaining anterior dentition, teeth #22 through 27. On examination, multiple teeth exhibit greater than 50 percent bone loss as demonstrated radiographically. Both #22 and #27 have existing PFM crowns, which have defective margins and recurrent decay. The treatment plan will involve removal of the remaining dentition #22 through #27, with placement of two implant fixtures at the same surgical event.

An immediate mandibular complete denture will be fabricated in advance of the scheduled surgery, and inserted with a soft reline on the day of surgery.

How would you code the removable prosthodontic procedures completed in advance of the scheduled surgery?

The correct coding for the removable prosthesis is:

D5140 immediate denture – mandible

There is no separate additional code for reline of the immediate denture in this case, since a reline of an immediate denture on the day of insertion is included in the parent code.

However, after the initial insertion, an immediate denture reverts to either a complete or partial denture. As such, any future reline would be coded as a separate and distinct procedure. In this case, a chairside reline at a future visit would be coded as:

D5731 reline complete mandibular denture (chairside)

CODING SCENARIO #3

Complete Denture Repair

A patient presents relating that they dropped their maxillary complete denture, resulting in fracture of the buccal flange along the right side including the area comprising the tuberosity. The denture is otherwise in good condition, and the flange is able to be accurately re-assembled and repaired with acrylic resin.

How would code this procedure?

D5512 repair broken complete denture base – maxillary

CODING SCENARIO #4

Reinforcement of the Denture Base for a Complete Denture

A patient with a history of fracture and repair of the denture base due to an opposing arch of natural dentition and a Class II jaw relationship presents for a new maxillary complete denture. In order to strengthen the denture base, a metal substructure is added to the palatal aspect of the new denture to enhance resistance to fracture during function.

How would code this procedure?

D5876 add metal substructure to acrylic complete denture (per arch)

Coding Q&A

1. **How is an immediate denture different than a partial or complete denture?**

   An immediate denture is a temporal code which only applies to the initial insertion of the denture prosthesis. Subsequent visits will code this prosthesis as either a partial or complete denture.

2. **How do I properly code refitting the denture base of an existing removable partial denture when additional teeth are added to this prosthesis?**

   If the entire denture base needs to be updated in an existing removable partial denture, meaning the borders of the edentulous area are developed to re-establish proper extension and contour, then the correct code for this procedure would be either **D5720 rebase maxillary partial denture**, or **D5721 rebase mandibular partial denture.**

   The code to add an additional tooth to this existing partial denture is **D5650 add tooth to existing partial denture**.

3. **How do I code for a partial denture that needs an adjustment and a repair?**

   A maxillary partial denture that has a broken clasp assembly typically requires both a repair and an adjustment once the new clasp assembly is joined to the framework. This should be coded as **D5630 repair or replace broken clasp – per tooth,** and **D5421 adjust partial denture – maxillary**.

4. **How is D5876 add metal substructure to acrylic full denture (per arch) intended to be used – is it applicable to fabrication of a new denture, or to the repair of an existing denture?**

   This procedure, added in CDT 2019, applies to fabrication of a new denture. It is not intended to be a repair procedure. According to the CDT Code Action Request's rationale for and technical description of the procedure as accepted by the Code Maintenance Committee, the procedure is an additional service when the prosthesis is being fabricated.

Summary

The procedure codes listed in this category describe services related to either a partial or complete denture. Keeping this concept in mind when coding for a procedure will simplify the decision making process to help delineate the correct code.

Contributor Biography

Terry M. Kelly, D.M.D. attended the University of Illinois and graduated from Southern Illinois School of Dental Medicine. He received a certificate in prosthodontics from Louisiana State University School of Dentistry, and completed a fellowship in maxillofacial prosthetics at M.D. Anderson Cancer Center. Dr. Kelly is certified by the American Board of Prosthodontics, has served on the Board of Directors of the American College of Prosthodontists. He is a past president of the American Academy of Maxillofacial Prosthetics, where he was part of the coding and reimbursement task force to establish CPT codes for maxillofacial prosthetic procedures. Dr. Kelly maintains a practice limited to implant dentistry with emphasis on full arch reconstruction.

Chapter 7.
D5900 – D5999
Maxillofacial Prosthetics

By Terri Bradley

Introduction

The CDT Code's Maxillofacial Prosthodontics category of service is a very unique section where the majority of the codes address procedures for devices often used for patients with cancer, trauma (such as gunshot wounds), cleft palate, etc. Due to the various medical conditions of these patients, the majority of the codes and services in this category would be submitted to medical carriers. There are, however, codes for procedures in this section that would be covered by dental carriers and not necessarily by medical carriers.

Key Definitions and Concepts

Splint: A prosthetic device which uses existing teeth or the alveolar process as points of anchorage to aid in the stabilization of broken bones (i.e., mandible, alveolar ridge) during healing. Splints are used to reestablish normal occlusion after trauma or procedures such as orthognathic surgery. These devices are stabilized by hard tissue.

Stent: A prosthetic device which is used to apply pressure to soft tissue to aid in healing and prevent scarring during healing. It can be used after surgery to aid in tissue closure and healing. Stents are often utilized for procedures post periodontal surgery, such as skin grafting.

Obturator: A prosthetic device which artificially replaces part of or all of the maxilla and associated teeth lost due to cancer, trauma or congenital defects. Obturators can be classified as interim, surgical and definitive.

Oral Prosthesis: An oral prosthesis is an artificial replacement which is either fixed or removable and aids in restoring normal form and function.

Changes to This Category

There are no changes to this category in CDT 2019.

Diagnosis Codes – ICD-10-CM

The CDT to ICD tables in Appendix 1 do not include guidance on linkages between Maxillofacial Prosthetics procedure codes and diagnosis codes as these tables focus on claims submitted to dental benefit plans. As noted in this chapter's introduction, Maxillofacial Prosthetics codes are often submitted to and covered by medical carriers, which do require providers to report diagnosis code(s) on the claim.

The following codes are a small sample that may be applicable. Please note that applicable ICD codes may be found in several sections of that code set, as indicated below.

C00 Neoplasms

C05.0 Malignant neoplasm of hard palate

C05.1 Malignant neoplasm of soft palate

G00 Diseases of the nervous system

G47.33 Obstructive Sleep Apnea

K00 Diseases of the digestive system

K11.7 Xerostomia

Q00 Congenital malformations, deformations and chromosomal abnormalities

Q37.1 Cleft hard palate with unilateral cleft lip

Q37.3 Cleft soft palate with unilateral cleft lip

Q37.5 Cleft hard and soft palate with unilateral cleft lip

Coding Scenarios

CODING SCENARIO #1

Implant Placement Guide

Four months after an extraction and socket preservation, a patient returns for endosteal implant placement at site #30. You fabricate a guide for the implant placement surgery. In the past, you have used **D5982 surgical stent** and you were recently told this is wrong.

How would you code this encounter?

The correct code to report for this scenario is **D6190 radiographic/surgical implant index, by report**. D5982 is not the appropriate code to report in this case as it is applicable when reporting a surgical stent to apply pressure to soft tissues to facilitate healing and prevent cicatrization or collapse.

CODING SCENARIO #2

Obturator for Cancer Patient

A patient was diagnosed with cancer involving the maxilla. You plan on fabricating an obturator for the patient. He already has an obturator that was delivered on the day of surgery.

What other obturator(s) might you fabricate for your patient and how would you code for this?

The provider can provide the patient with an interim (D5936) and definitive obturator (D5932) or they can modify the surgical obturator (D5933) and provide a definitive one. In that case, the final definitive obturator (D5932) would be fabricated once healing is complete.

CODING SCENARIO #3

Appliance for Patient Undergoing Radiation Therapy

Your patient is diagnosed with squamous cell carcinoma and is scheduled to undergo radiation therapy. In order to best protect the unaffected tongue and oral mucosa, you decide to fabricate an oral appliance.

How would you code this?

You would use D5984 radiation shield.

CODING SCENARIO #4

Protecting Dentition During Cancer Treatment

A patient was recently diagnosed with cancer of the tongue and will be undergoing radiation therapy in the very near future. The patient's oncologist suggested the patient see you to discuss ways to protect the dentition during cancer therapy. The doctor recommends fluoride trays for the patient.

How would you code this?

D5986 fluoride gel carrier
Synonymous terminology: fluoride applicator. A prosthesis, which covers the teeth in either dental arch and is used daily to apply topical fluoride in close proximity to tooth enamel and dentin for several minutes daily.

CODING SCENARIO #5

Snoring and Treatment Appliances

A patient comes in stating that his wife complained his snoring is so loud at night that some nights she sleeps in the other room. He has seen his medical doctor and has been told that he does not have obstructive sleep apnea; he is just a loud snorer and his snoring seems to be worse after a high stress day. The doctor fabricates a snore guard for the patient.

How would you code for this?

Many people are unaware that the Maxillofacial Prosthetics category includes a number of non-orthodontic treatment appliances. However, there is not a specific code for the snore guard. Since such an appliance is similar to other appliances in the Maxillofacial Prosthetics category, it would be appropriate to use this code:

D5999 unspecified maxillofacial prosthesis, by report

CODING SCENARIO #6

Mouth Lesions

A 50-year-old woman comes to the office stating that she has painful lesions in her mouth. Upon clinical inspection, it is noted that the tissue is erythematous and the lesions look erosive in nature, and there are some bullae present. You suspect that the patient has pemphigus vulgaris. The patient states that the lesions have been there for four days and that she has been self-treating with salt water rinses. You prescribe topical steroid for the lesions and arrange for the lab to create a medicament carrier that will cover the affected areas.

How would you code this?

D5991 vesiculobullous disease medicament carriers
A custom fabricated carrier the covers the teeth and alveolar mucosa, or alveolar mucosa alone, and is used to deliver prescription medicaments for treatment of immunologically mediated vesiculobullous diseases

CODING SCENARIO #7

Malignant Neoplasm of the Hard Palate

Your patient has been diagnosed with a malignant neoplasm of the hard palate. Prior to surgery, you fabricate a surgical obturator to be placed after the removal of the neoplasm. The patient also receives radiation treatment, for which you fabricate a radiation shield. After the surgery, the plan is to fabricate both an interim and definitive prosthesis. However, due to the fit of the surgical obturator, an interim prosthesis is not needed by the patient and instead only the definitive prosthesis is created.

How would you code this?

D5984 radiation shield

D5931 obturator prosthesis surgical (CPT 21076)

D5932 obturator prosthesis, definitive (CPT 21080)

If the surgical obturator is to be modified prior to placement of a definitive obturator, the code would be:

D5992 adjust maxillofacial prosthetic appliance, by report

Maintenance of the obturator would be coded as:

D5993 maintenance and cleaning of a maxillofacial prosthesis (extra- or intra-oral) other than required by adjustments, by report

Coding Q&A

1. **I am a maxillofacial prosthodontist working in a large academic setting. The patients I am treating have some pretty significant medical conditions. What are the codes I would use to bill to a dental carrier and a medical carrier for the surgical, interim and definitive obturator prosthesis?**

   Surgical obturator: CDT code is **D5931**; CPT code is **21076**

   Interim obturator prosthesis: CDT code is **D5936**; CPT code is **21079**

   Definitive obturator prosthesis: CDT code is **D5932**; CPT code is **21080**

   If the claim is being filed with the patient's medical benefit plan using the appropriate (not dental) claim format the following ICD-10 code is appropriate:

   ICD-10: C05.0 Malignant neoplasm of the hard palate

2. **What is the difference between a surgical, interim and definitive obturator? The terms are so confusing!**

   A surgical obturator is created and used during surgery and immediately post-operatively. The interim prosthesis is used for the duration of the healing, which can be anywhere from two to six months. After about six months, the definitive prosthesis is given to the patient, and it may last for many years.

3. **A patient has an obturator fabricated pre-operatively for placement immediately after a tumor removal surgery. Due to the excellent fit and comfort of this obturator, the patient decides they do not want another until the final prosthesis is fabricated. How would you code this?**

   You would use **D5993 obturator prosthesis, modification**.

4. **Are obturators used only for cancer patients?**

   No, obturators can be used for patients with a various medical conditions. Patients with palatal perforations due to infection, disease, recreational drug use, or cleft palate may require an obturator as part of their treatment. Not all patients will require a definitive obturator. Some may need a surgical or interim obturator while receiving treatment or in between reconstructive surgeries.

5. **I'm still a little confused about the different types of obturators and when they're used. Can you go into more detail?**

   Surgical obturators (D5931) are delivered to the patient on the date of surgery. It may not fit exactly and will likely require some adjustment. An interim obturator is intended to be used prior to the fabrication of a definitive obturator during the healing period. The patient will likely have this for a number of months. Sometimes, if the fit is good, a patient will opt to have their surgical obturator modified rather than have an interim obturator fabricated. A definitive obturator is fabricated after healing has occurred. It is designed to be the patient's "final" obturator, though if the patient has it for a number of years it will likely need to be replaced.

6. **What is the difference between a radiation shield and a radiation carrier?**

   The shield protects the tissues from radiation and the carrier is used for applying radiation to the area.

7. **What is the difference between a fluoride gel carrier (D5986) and a periodontal medicament carrier with peripheral seal-laboratory processed (D5994)?**

   A fluoride gel carrier is used for application of topic fluoride only and it only covers the teeth.

   The periodontal medicament carrier, however, covers both the teeth and the alveolar mucosa. It is used to deliver medications to tissues (gingiva), membranes (alveolar mucosa), and into periodontal pockets.

8. **In dental coding, is there a separate code for a snoring appliance versus an appliance for patients with sleep apnea?**

   There is not a specific CDT code for either appliance. The best choice of code is to use **D5999 unspecified maxillofacial prosthesis, by report**. For medical coding, it is important to remember that while many patients with sleep apnea do snore, not all patients who snore have sleep apnea and the medical codes for the various appliances are very different. Diagnosis of obstructive sleep apnea is required to bill for an OSA appliance to a medical carrier.

9. Is a sleep study required before I can code for a sleep apnea appliance?

There is no specific code for a sleep apnea appliance, so you would use:

D5999 unspecified maxillofacial prosthesis, by report

The patient will need to have a formal diagnosis of obstructive sleep apnea. This usually includes a sleep study.

If you file a claim with the patient's medical benefit plan the following codes are applicable:

HCPCS procedure – E0486 oral device/appliance used to reduce upper airway collapsibility, adjustable or non-adjustable, custom fabricated, includes fitting and adjustment

ICD-10 diagnosis – G47.33 Obstructive Sleep Apnea

10. What is a vesiculobullous disease?

A vesiculobullous disease is one in which vesicles and bullae are both present. Both are fluid filled lesions and bullae are larger than vesicles. These disorders can be considered mucocutaneous diseases due to their involvement in the skin and the mucous membranes of the oral cavity.

11. What are some examples of vesiculobullous diseases?

Examples of vesiculobullous diseases include:
- Paraneoplastic pemphigus
- Pemphigus vulgaris
- Bullous pemphigoid
- Erythema multiforme
- Herpes Simplex

12. A patient requires medication to be delivered to soft tissue areas in the oral cavity due to painful ulcerated lesions. Which prosthesis would be delivered and how would it be coded?

The patient would require a disease medicament carrier, not a periodontal medicament carrier, as a seal is not required. The applicable procedure is documented with CDT code **D5991 vesiculobullous disease medicament carrier**.

13. **Can I use the "periodontal medicament carrier" and "vesiculobullous disease medicament carrier" codes on the same patient? Are these codes somewhat interchangeable?**

These two codes are not interchangeable. While both are used to describe medicament carriers, the need for these two appliances are quite different. **D5991 vesiculobullous disease medicament carrier** can only be used for patients who have a vesiculobullous disease. The periodontal medicament carrier (**D5994**) is used primarily to treat periodontal disease and deliver medications targeted at the pathogens that cause various periodontal diseases. These appliances are treating two different disease processes, D5994 is used to treat diseases that are periodontal in nature while D5991 is used to treat mucocutaneous diseases involving mucous membranes and skin.

14. **Can D5994 be used for patients who have vesiculobullous diseases or for cancer patients who need fluoride delivered?**

No, this code can only be used for periodontal medicaments. Its use is aimed at delivering medication to target pathogens that cause periodontal disease. The pathogens that cause perio disease are not the same as the ones that cause vesiculobullous diseases and so D5991 should be used instead. For patients requiring fluoride, D5986 should be used. It is limited to intraoral trays fabricated solely for the delivery of fluoride.

Summary

Due to the severity of the medical condition of so many of the patients seen by maxillofacial prosthodontists (i.e., cancer, gunshot wound, cleft, ameloblastoma, etc.), the majority of the procedures will be billed to medical carriers. Thus, it is important to ensure that you are using the proper CPT code if there is one (there are not always individual CPT codes for all CDT codes) when coding. If there is no specific CPT code, you may bill the medical carrier using the CDT code.

The other pitfall to coding for these procedures for the coder (not necessarily the provider) is a clear understanding of what is actually happening and why is the prosthesis being fabricated in the first place. The definitions are very specific and it is necessary to understand the nuances and differences between them.

Contributor Biography

Terri Bradley is the owner of Terri Bradley Consulting and OMS Billing Solutions. With a hands-on background spanning more than 30 years, Terri is a practice management expert devoted to her clients. She is highly sought after for speaking engagements offering medical/dental/OMS coding and billing workshops across the country. Her publications include the Fonseca Oral and Maxillofacial Surgery textbook chapter (Volume III, released fall 2017) and Dictations and Coding in Oral and Maxillofacial Surgery.

Chapter 8.
D6000 – D6199
Implant Services

By Linda Vidone, D.M.D.

Introduction

The CDT Code's Implant Services category is somewhat unique compared to other categories of service because it includes separate entries for procedures that address:

- Surgical placement of the implant post (or body or fixture)
- Placement of connecting components when needed
- The final prosthetic restoration (single crowns, bridges or dentures)

Once these three basic concepts of implant procedures (addressed in greater detail below) are understood, it will become less challenging and even easy to select the appropriate CDT Code to document the procedures performed.

Key Definitions and Concepts

Basic Implant

This image illustrates all components of a single implant. Please note that the connecting element (abutment) may not be present in all cases. The dentist's clinical decision-making determines whether the implant crown will be supported and retained by an intermediary abutment, or if it may be placed directly on the implant body.

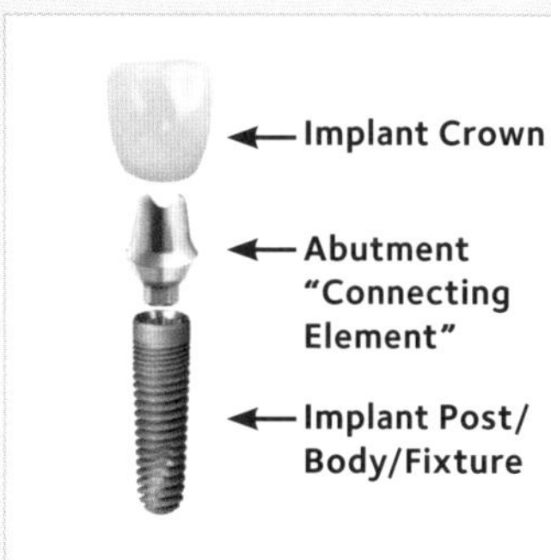

Image courtesy of Glidewell Laboratories

Implant Post/Body/Fixture

The two most common types of implant posts are endosteal and mini implants. The size and type of implant fixture determines the proper code to document the surgical implant placement procedure.

Surgical Placement of an Implant Body: Endosteal Implant (D6010): Placement of full-sized implant fixture into the jawbone.

Surgical Placement of Mini-Implant (D6013): Placement of mini-implant fixture into the jawbone. These are smaller in diameter than full-sized implants, yet are still considered permanent. Typically used to support removable prostheses.

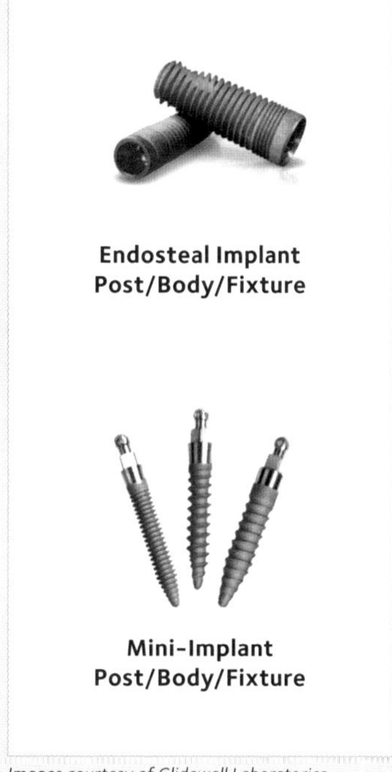

Images courtesy of Glidewell Laboratories

Connecting Elements for Implant Crowns and Implant Retainer Crowns

Abutments, both prefabricated (D6056) and custom (D6057), are the "connecting elements" that are placed, when needed, between the implant post and the restorative crown (definitive prosthesis) or retainer crown (for a fixed partial denture). Abutments are not always needed, but when placed are reported separately from the from the crown restoration.

Prefabricated Abutment (D6056): A manufactured component. The procedure includes modification and placement.

Custom Abutment (D6057): Created by a laboratory for a specific individual, usually if there are aesthetic concerns. The procedure includes placement. Custom abutments are custom cast or CAD/CAM milled.

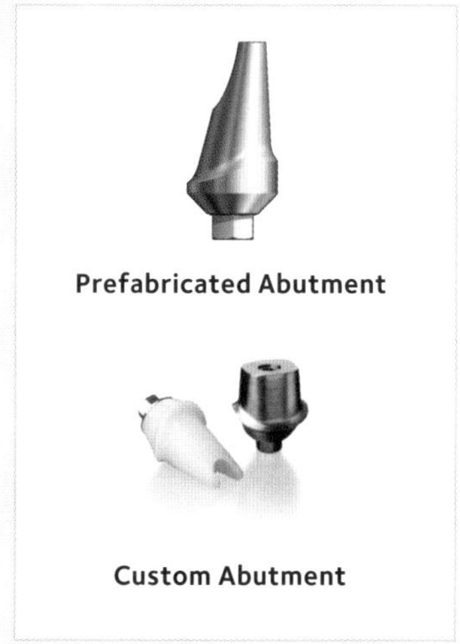

Images courtesy of Glidewell Laboratories

Connecting Elements for Implant Dentures

Semi-precision Attachment Abutment (D6052): An attachment which involves placement of the prefabricated abutment to the implant post (full sized) and includes the luting of the keeper assembly (male attachment) into the overdenture.

Connecting Bar – Implant Supported or Abutment Supported (D6055): A device to help stabilize prostheses. Attaches to abutments or directly to the implants themselves to make the prosthesis more secure. Hader® and Dolder® are two types of connecting bars that can be designed to use other types of retentive mechanisms, such as semi-precision attachments. The entire bar is reported as a single unit; however an abutment would be documented for each implant that supports the connecting bar.

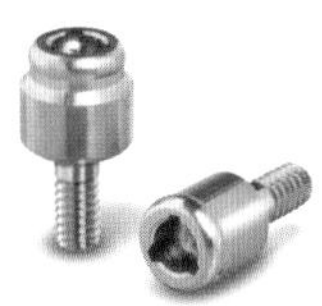

Semi-precision Attachment Abutment

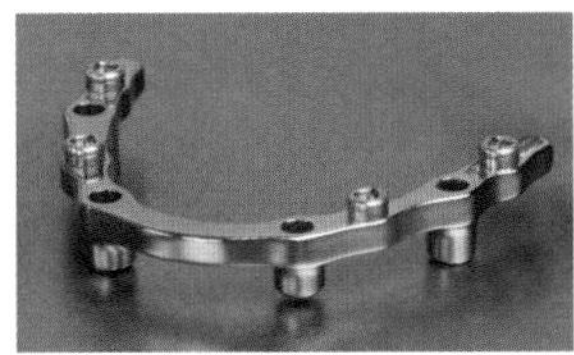

Connecting Bar – Implant Supported or Abutment Supported

Image courtesy of Glidewell Laboratories

Implant Prosthesis (Includes Single Crowns, Fixed Bridges and Dentures)

There are two types of single unit implant crowns – abutment supported and Implant supported. Selection of the appropriate crown procedure code is determined by the type of material used for the crown, and the type of attachment.

Most of us are familiar with the type of material used (porcelain, metal, etc.). However, there is some confusion when it comes to the type of attachment system used-abutment or implant supported.

Note: Both abutment supported and implant supported crowns are either cemented or screw retained, but neither method is a determining factor in code selection.

Abutment Supported Single Unit Crowns (D6058-D6064, D6094): These are crowns that are attached to an abutment (D6056 or D6057), not directly to the implant post. The applicable abutment procedure code is submitted with the applicable single unit crown procedure code. This is the most common type of implant crown.

Implant Supported Single Unit Crowns (D6065-D6067): Implant crowns are attached directly to the implant post (one-piece retained crown); *No abutment is used with this type crown.*

Single Unit Crowns

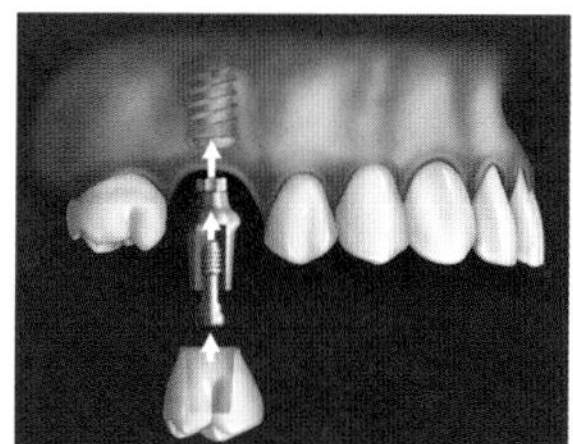

Abutment

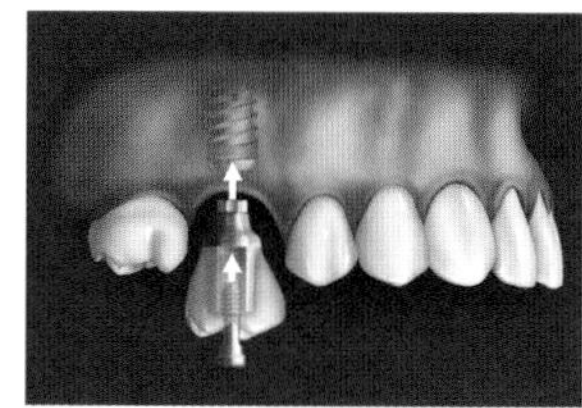

No abutment

Image courtesy of Glidewell Laboratories

Implant Supported Fixed Partial Dentures (Implant Bridges)

There are two types of implant retainer crowns: abutment supported and implant supported. Selection of the appropriate retainer crown procedure code is based on the same criteria used for single implant crowns: the type of material used and the method of attachment.

Note: Both abutment supported and implant supported retainer crowns are either cemented or screw retained, and neither method is a determining factor in code selection.

Abutment Supported Retainer Crowns (D6068–D6074 and D6194): These are retainer crowns that are attached to an abutment (D6056 or D6057), not directly to the implant post. The applicable abutment procedure code is submitted with the applicable retainer crown procedure code.

Implant Supported Retainer Crowns (D6075-D6077): Implant retainer crowns are attached directly to the implant post. *No abutment is used with this type crown.*

Implant/Abutment Supported Dentures

There are two types of implant or abutment supported dentures: removable and fixed (also known as hybrid). Implant dentures, unlike single unit crowns and retainer crowns, are NOT determined by the type of attachment system.

Denture procedure code selection is determined by two factors:

- Is the denture replacing a full or partial complement of teeth?
- Will the patient be able to remove the denture by themselves, or is assistance needed from the dentist or dental staff?

If the patient is able to remove the denture by themselves, it is a removable implant denture. If the patient is unable to remove the denture and requires the assistance of dentist or dental staff, then the denture is a fixed implant denture.

Although a fixed implant bridge and fixed implant denture appear similar, the denture's supporting implant locations do not have a specific relationship to the missing natural teeth. This is why a fixed implant denture is referred to as a "hybrid" denture.

Implant/Abutment Supported Removable Dentures: Overdentures are supported by implants; the patient is able remove them. These dentures typically have prefabricated abutments placed, a connecting bar, and a precision or semi-precision attachment. (Note these components are not included in the denture and should all be submitted as separate procedures.) Codes for removable complete dentures are D6110 and D6111; codes for removable partials are D6112 and D6113.

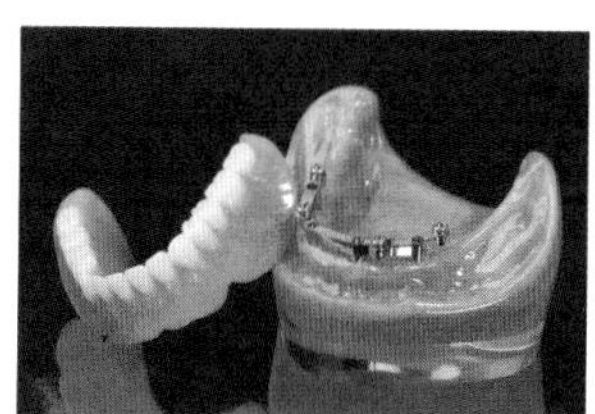

Implant/abutment supported removable dentures

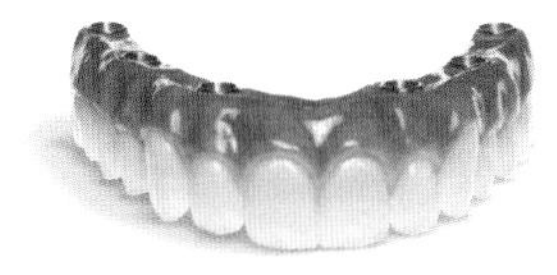

Hybrid dentures

Image courtesy of Glidewell Laboratories

Implant/Abutment Supported Fixed (Hybrid) Dentures: Implant dentures that the patient cannot remove and are either screwed directly on the implant or connected via abutments. (Note abutments are not included in the denture and when used should be submitted as separate procedures.) Codes for fixed complete dentures (dentures that replace all missing teeth) are D6114 and D6115. Typically four to eight implants are utilized and are not in absolute tooth positions. Codes for fixed partials are D6116 and D6117.

Changes to This Category

There are no changes to this category in CDT 2019.

Abutment vs. Retainer

When implant procedures were first introduced in CDT-1 (effective January 1, 1990), confusion arose over the term abutment, a word with different meanings within the Implants category of service and within the Prosthodontics category of service. For Implants, "abutment" was associated with the piece that connected the implant body with the restorative prosthesis. In Prosthodontics, the term was used to describe a supporting (anchor) tooth in a fixed bridge.

The current and continuing usage for the term "abutment" applies only to the piece that connects the implant body with the restorative prosthesis. "Retainer" is the term solely used to describe the anchor tooth (natural or prosthetic) for a fixed partial denture.

Diagnosis Codes – ICD-10-CM

The CDT to ICD tables in Appendix 1 provide appropriate guidance on linkages between Implant Services procedure codes and diagnosis codes.

In some cases dental implants maybe covered by the patient's medial carrier. Clear communication to the medical carrier is needed to explain the purpose of the implant procedure. This communication is also aided by using the CDT-ICD tables in Appendix 1 to select a diagnosis applicable to the patient's conditions and symptoms.

Notes:

- Claims against a patient's medical benefit plan uses the AMA's CPT procedure codes on the medical claim format.
- Medical carriers may benefit for the implant placement and necessary bone grafting, but the final restorative prosthesis is typically never a benefit.

A sample of CPT codes for implant placement and bone grafting are in the following tables:

Surgical Placement and Removal of Dental Implants	
Code	**Nomenclature**
20670	Removal of implant, superficial
20680	Removal of implant, deep
21248	Reconstruction of maxilla/mandible endosteal implant, partial (1-3 per jaw)
21249	Reconstruction of maxilla/mandible endosteal implant, complete (4-6 per jaw)
21085	Diagnostic/surgical stent
Bone Grafts	
Code	**Nomenclature**
21210	Graft, bone, nasal, maxillary, or malar areas (includes obtaining graft)
21215	Graft, bone, mandibular areas (includes obtaining graft)
0232T	Platelet rich plasma
41899	Nonspecific code (Used for Guided Tissue Regeneration)

CODING SCENARIO #1

Abutment Supported Porcelain Implant Crown Tooth #7

The patient is 30 years old with a long history of dental treatment on #7. She got hit by a ball in her mouth when she was 14 years old. The only tooth affected was #7. She had a root canal with a post and core crown placed at the time of the accident. When she was 22 years old, she had retreatment of the root canal, apicoectomy, and a new post and core crown.

The tooth is now re-infected and the dentist suspects a vertical fracture. She has class 2 mobility with 7 mm pocket on the buccal, thus having a poor prognosis. The adjacent teeth are perfectly healthy with no restorations nor do they need restorations. After all options were discussed, the patient chose the best option which was a single tooth implant.

What codes would be used to document services of the treatment plan leading to the single tooth implant?

Extraction of #7 with Ridge Preservation and Insertion of a "Flipper"

D7210 extraction, erupted tooth requiring removal of bone and/or sectioning of tooth

D7953 bone replacement graft for ridge preservation – per site

Notes:

- Bone in this area is thin, therefore it is imperative that the ridge be preserved.
- This procedure is also referred to as "socket preservation" with the placed in the extraction site at the time of the extraction to preserve the size and shape of the bone.

D4266 guided tissue regeneration – resorbable barrier, per site

Note: The D7953 procedure does not include placement of a barrier membrane to prevent tissue from invading the bone graft site and there is no separate code for a membrane with ridge preservation. D4266 is used to document placement of the barrier membrane.

D5820 interim partial denture (maxillary)

Note: D5820 is the "flipper" procedure.

Implant Placement Surgery and Second Stage Surgery

Note: The implant post is surgically placed and followed by second stage surgery six months later.

D6010 surgical placement of implant body: endosteal implant

D6011 second stage surgery

Final Restoration – Custom Abutment and Abutment Supported Porcelain Crown

Note: In this case, esthetics were a concern. A custom abutment was placed due to angulation concerns and final material chosen was porcelain since the patient has a high smile line.

D6057 custom abutment placed

D6058 abutment supported porcelain/ceramic crown

CODING SCENARIO #2

Implant Supported Mandibular Denture for an Edentulous Patient

The patient has worn a complete mandibular denture for over 10 years with an occasional reline. The most recent reline was two years ago. Before this there were no problems with fit or retention, but since the last reline the patient has been using an adhesive to glue in the denture with limited success. The patient is also edentulous on the maxillary, but is happy with her denture. The patient had previously declined a recommendation to replace the denture with implants and fabricate an overdenture over the implant. Now the patient has agreed to implant treatment.

What codes would be used to document services delivered as the treatment progressed?

Initial Services

Since the patient has been edentulous for over ten years, a cone beam CT scan was necessary to evaluate the mandibular jaw bone dimensions. This enables an assessment to determine whether bone augmentation is needed prior to implant placement. A surgical stent was made and used during radiographic exposure for treatment planning and will be used again during implant placement.

D0365 cone beam CT capture and interpretation with limited field of view of one full dental arch – mandible

D6190 radiographic/surgical implant index, by report

Implant Post Placement

The cone beam image revealed there was enough bone to place two implants in positions of teeth #22 and 27. However, after placing the implant bodies a few threads were exposed, so a bone graft and membrane were also necessary.

D6010 surgical placement of implant body: endosteal implant

Note: Report D6010 twice as two implant bodies were placed, one for #22 and the second for #27.

D6104 bone graft at the time of implant placement

Note: The bone graft procedure (D6104) does not include placement of a barrier membrane and there is no separate code for membranes with implant bone grafts. Use one of the following codes, as applicable, to report barrier membrane placement.

D4266 guided tissue regeneration – resorbable barrier, per site

D4267 guided tissue regeneration – non-resorbable barrier, per site (includes membrane removal)

Second Stage Surgery and Placement of the Restorative Prosthesis

The patient will continue to wear her existing denture as the implants heal. After the implants have successfully integrated, the next step is to begin the restorative treatment. Second stage surgery is followed by placement of semi-precision attachments. A newly fabricated mandibular complete overdenture is inserted.

These procedures are documented as follows:

D6011 second stage surgery

Note: Report D6011 twice as the procedure is required for each of the two implant bodies placed.

D6052 semi-precision attachment abutment

Note: Report D6052 twice as the procedure is required for each of the two implant bodies placed.

D6111 implant/abutment supported removable denture for edentulous arch – mandibular

Note: This code is used for removable complete dentures that are either directly supported by the implant body, or by the abutments placed on the implant body.

Replacement of Semi-Precision Attachment Male Component

The patient is made aware that it is normal for the attachment's male components to wear over time, and will periodically need replacement. This future procedure is documented with the following CDT code.

D6091 replacement of semi-precision or precision attachment of implant/abutment supported prosthesis, per attachment

CODING SCENARIO #3

Implant Supported Maxillary Fixed Complete Denture

The patient in scenario two was so happy with the results of her lower denture she would now like implants on her maxilla. The final prostheses for this arch will be an abutment supported fixed complete denture.

What codes would be used to document services delivered as the treatment progressed?

Initial Services

Since the patient has low sinuses a cone beam scan was necessary to evaluate their exact location as well as the jaw bone dimensions. This enables an assessment to determine whether sinus elevation and bone augmentation is needed prior to implant placement. A surgical stent was made and used during radiographic exposure for treatment planning and will be used again during implant placement.

D0365 cone beam CT capture and interpretation with limited field of view of one full dental arch-mandible

D6190 radiographic/surgical implant index, by report

Implant Post Placement and Sinus Elevation

The restorative dentist would like six implants placed since the final restoration will be a fixed denture. The cone beam image revealed there was enough bone in areas of teeth #7 and 10 however in areas of #3, 5, 12, and 14 sinus elevation will be needed. Note the patients existing denture will be utilized after implant placement and sinus elevation.

D6010 surgical placement of implant body: endosteal implant

Note: Report D6010 six times since six implant bodies were placed, one for #3, 5, 7, 10, 12 and 14.

D7951 sinus augmentation with bone or bone substitutes via a lateral open approach

D7952 sinus augmentation via a vertical approach

Note: Report the appropriate sinus elevation twice – once on the right side and once on the left and both these procedures include obtaining the bone or bone substitutes.

Second Stage Surgery and Placement Interim Prosthesis and Final Prosthetic

After three to six months of osseointegration, implants are uncovered and an interim prosthesis is fabricated. An interim prosthesis was fabricated to evaluate the patient's esthetic and functional needs as well as soft tissue healing, and assist with design of the definitive prosthesis. After healing is complete a newly fabricated implant supported fixed complete denture is inserted.

These procedures are documented as follows:

D6011 second stage surgery

Note: Report D6011 six times as the procedure is required for each of the six implant bodies placed.

D6119 implant/abutment supported interim fixed denture for edentulous arch-maxillary

Note: D6119 is used during the healing prior to fabrication and placement of permanent prosthetic.

D6114 implant/abutment supported fixed denture for edentulous arch-maxillary

Note: This code is used for fixed complete dentures that are either directly supported by the implant body, or by the abutments placed on the implant body.

CODING SCENARIO #4

Removal of a Broken Implant Retaining Screw

Five years ago a dentist replaced tooth #19 with an implant post that successfully osseointegrated and an implant supported crown. The patient came in for an emergency since he felt "something was loose." The radiograph image shows the post is still osseointegrated with no bone loss. However, the implant retaining screw is broken.

How do you code for this visit?

D0140 limited oral evaluation

D0220 intraoral – periapical first radiographic image

D6096 remove broken implant retaining screw

This procedure assumes the implant retaining screw is broken and the fragments are remaining in the body of the implant as well as the implant retained crown. This code is only submitted when removing the screw cannot be performed using standard and conventional techniques for removal. When submitting to a dental plan, always submit a narrative with any supporting documentation.

CODING SCENARIO #5

Tightening of an Implant Screw

A dentist placed a screw retained porcelain fused to metal implant crown on tooth #12 two years ago. Today the patient was returning for a cleaning, exam and four bitewings. The patient had no concerns in her mouth, but the hygienist noticed that the implant screw was loose and needed to be tightened. After the prophy was completed, radiographs were taken. The dentist performed a periodontic exam, which showed that the screw was slightly loose, and proceeded to tighten the implant screw.

How would you code for this visit?

D1110 prophylaxis – adult

D0274 bitewings – four radiographic images

D0120 periodic oral evaluation

There is no separate code for tightening for tightening an implant retaining screw. This service may be reported with the unspecified implant services code D6199 accompanied by a detailed narrative.

Note: The Code Maintenance Committee considers tightening loose screws as inclusive to the implant maintenance procedure (D6080), which was not performed in this scenario.

CODING SCENARIO #6

Cantilever Implant

The patient desperately wants implants. She presented with missing #4 and 5 premolars. Her previous dentist wanted to place two implants in each location since #3 and 6 are healthy, caries-free teeth. She agreed with the treatment plan. However, after he reviewed the cone beam, he stated that a sinus elevation must be performed to place tooth #4. The patient refused the sinus elevation due to a lengthy history of sinus infections.

She arrives at the office of another dentist for a second opinion. She wants to see if the other dentist could place the implants without the sinus elevation. Upon review of the cone beam image from the previous dentist, the second dentist agrees that only the tooth #5 implant could be placed without the sinus elevation. The proposed treatment from the second dentist is one surgical implant on tooth #5 with a pontic and implant crown on teeth #4 and 5 respectively. The second dentist knows she will be cantilevering tooth #4 off tooth #5.

What code reports this cantilever crown # 5 which will be connected on an implant?

D6010 surgical implant placement of implant body (tooth #5)

D6076 implant supported retainer for porcelain fused to metal FPD (tooth #5)

D6240 pontic-porcelain fused to high noble metal (tooth #4)

A cantilever (fixed) bridge on a natural tooth would be submitted as D62XX pontic plus D67XX retainer crown. For the implant situation, you could still use the pontic codes D62XX, but would also use the implant retainer codes based on the material used and the method of attachment (D6068-D6077 and D6194).

Remember that the pontic codes, found in the Fixed Prosthodontic category of the CDT Code, can be used with all bridges whether the bridge is on natural teeth or implants. All pontic codes (D6205-D6253) can be used with either an abutment or implant supported bridge. Be sure the implant crown retainer material is consistent with the pontic material.

CODING SCENARIO #7

Implant/Abutment Supported Interim Fixed Denture for Edentulous Arch – Maxilla

A patient is completely edentulous on his upper jaw and he choose implants as an option. The implants will not be in relative tooth positions since the surgeon will place the implants were the ridge is sufficient. The final prosthesis will be a complete abutment supported fixed denture (a hybrid prosthesis). The dentist will be placing abutments and an interim fixed denture for this patient on the day of surgery so the patient doesn't have to go without teeth.

How do you code for the interim fixed denture?

D6119 Implant/abutment supported interim fixed denture for edentulous arch-maxillary

Since the case is in the maxillary arch, the correct code is D6119. The implant abutments (interim D6051, prefabricated D6056, or custom D6057) should be reported separately. If the denture will not be connected to the implants and is merely a removable denture, then the correct code is interim complete (removable) mandibular D5811.

CODING SCENARIO #8

Implant Overdenture – Mandibular

A 45-year-old patient has worn a complete mandibular denture for five years since she lost her teeth due to periodontal disease. She would like a more stable denture. Since her finances are limited, she opted for an overdenture which will be supported by two mini-implants in location of teeth #22 and 27. She will utilize her current denture as a temporary denture while the implants heal, but ultimately wants a new overdenture.

What codes should the dentist submit for the mini implants and the overdenture?

D6013 **surgical placement of mini implant** (#22 and 27)

D6111 **implant/abutment supported removable denture for edentulous arch-mandibular** (mandibular implant overdenture)

D6052 **semi-precision attachment abutments** (#22 and 27)

The D6052 procedure includes the keeper assembly which is luted in the denture.

CODING SCENARIO #9

Cervitec Gel Application Around an Implant to Treat Gingivitis

A dentist placed an implant and implant supported crown on tooth #6 five years ago. The implant is stable and radiographs show no bone loss around the implant fixture. The patient has very good oral hygiene. However, every time the patient presents for periodontal maintenance the tissue around the implant is inflamed. The dentist recently took a course and learned about a product she can apply to the tissue to treat this type of tissue inflammation around the implant. She purchased the material and will apply the gel on the gingival tissue and the implant restoration.

How would you code this procedure?

D6199 **unspecified implant procedure, by report**

Currently there is no CDT code to support application of the material that reduces tissue inflammation.

Coding Q&A

1. **My patient does not have implant coverage, but does have crown coverage. Would I be able to use the code D2740 instead of D6065 to report an implant supported porcelain/ceramic crown?**

   No. If implants are not a covered benefit under the patient's benefits, reporting D2740 is misrepresenting a service to gain insurance reimbursement. You must report the procedure performed (D6065) regardless of insurance reimbursement. This statement also applies for retainer crowns. Reporting Implant retainer crowns (D60XX) as retainer crowns on natural teeth (D67XX) to gain insurance reimbursement is also misrepresenting a service.

   Note: Even though you may be submitting the implant crowns appropriately, occasionally benefit plans may reimburse the implant crown as an alternate benefit of a natural tooth crown.

2. **I submitted a claim to my patient's dental insurance carrier for two implant procedures for tooth #12: D6066 implant supported porcelain fused to metal crown and D6056 prefabricated abutment. The carrier has not reimbursed procedures, stating "Implant abutments must be submitted with an abutment supported prosthetics. Please resubmit with the appropriate codes." What do I do?**

   The insurance carrier is correct. When you are using an abutment (either D6056 or D6057), this must be followed by an abutment-supported prosthesis. In your case, since you are using an abutment, the correct code is **D6059 abutment supported porcelain fused to metal crown**. The code D6066 is an implant supported crown and does not require an abutment.

3. **What is the difference between a temporary anchorage device (TAD) (D7292, D7293 or D7294) and a mini implant (D6013)?**

   Although both TADs and mini implants look similar, a TAD is typically smaller, has an area for orthodontic wire, is used for orthodontic anchorage or as part of orthodontic treatment, and is removed after a period of time. A mini implant (D6013) is not typically removed and usually supports a removable denture.

4. **My patient is having endosteal implants placed for a complete implant supported denture. The dentist will fabricate a stent-like appliance for the surgeon to be sure the implants are placed exactly where the dentist needs them. Would the appliance be documented as D5982 surgical stent, D5988 surgical splint or D6190 radiographic/surgical implant index, by report?**

   The correct code is:

   D6190 radiographic/surgical implant index, by report
   An appliance, designed to relate osteotomy or fixture position to existing anatomic structures, to be utilized during radiographic exposure for treatment planning and/or during osteotomy creation for fixture installation.

   D5982 surgical stent is not correct because a stent is an appliance that applies pressure to soft tissues to facilitate healing and prevent collapse of soft tissue.

   D5988 surgical stent uses existing teeth and/or alveolar processes as points of anchorage to assist in stabilization and immobilization of broken bones during healing.

5. **I noticed there are no pontic codes in the CDT Code's Implant Services category. When reporting a fixed partial denture placed on implants, how do I report the pontic?**

   Pontic codes, found in the Fixed Prosthodontic category of the CDT Code, can be used with all bridges whether the bridge is on natural teeth or implants. All pontic codes (**D6205–D6253**) can be used with either an abutment or implant supported bridge. Be sure the implant crown retainer material is consistent with the pontic material.

6. **I placed an implant on tooth #30 two years ago. The patient has since developed peri-implantitis. There is radiographic evidence of bone loss only on the mesial aspect, so I am confident this can successfully be treated with bone grafting. Would the osseous surgery procedure be documented with D4261, and the bone graft documented with D4263?**

No, the D426x procedure codes are not appropriate for documenting surgical repairs and bone grafting in conjunction with implants. The correct codes in this situation are:

D6102 debridement and osseous contouring of a peri-implant defect or defects surrounding a single implant and includes surface cleaning of exposed implant surfaces, including flap entry and closure

D6103 bone graft for repair of peri-implant defect – does not include flap entry and closure

Placement of a barrier membrane or biologic materials to aid in osseous regeneration are reported separately.

7. **The current CDT manual does not include the following entry: "D6020 abutment placement or substitution: endosteal implant." What code should I use now to document this procedure?**

There were concurrent changes in CDT 2005 that included deletion of D6020 and revision to the implant abutment codes (D6056-D6057). These revisions clarified that the abutment procedures included placement. The current codes and their nomenclatures follow:

D6056 prefabricated abutment – includes modification and placement

D6057 custom fabricated abutment – includes placement

8. **We have several patients that have implant supported mandibular complete dentures. However, they have natural teeth in their maxillary arch. What procedure code would be used to report cleaning of the implants and can this code be submitted with a prophy (D1110) and a periodic oral evaluation (D0120)?**

The correct code in this situation is:

D6080 implant maintenance procedures when prostheses are removed and reinserted, including cleansing of prostheses and abutments

This procedure includes active debriding of the implant(s) and examination of all aspects of the implant system(s), including the occlusion and stability of the superstructure. The patient is also instructed in thorough daily cleansing of the implant(s). This is not a per implant code, it is for implant supported fixed prostheses (hybrid or implant supported bridge).

Implant maintenance (D6080) can be submitted for the same date of service that the patient receives a prophylaxis (D1110) or periodontal maintenance (D4910), because the implant maintenance procedure does not include services rendered to natural teeth in the patient's mouth. A periodic oral evaluation D0120 can also be submitted on this date of service.

However, when both the D6080 and D1110 are performed on the same date of service some dental benefit plan limitations and exclusions provisions may, for claim adjudication, the dental plan may consider D6080 to be inclusive in the D1110 (or D4910) and D0120 procedure and not provide additional reimbursement.

9. **I placed provisional crowns on three implants to allow time for healing which should take in about six months. There are provisional crowns in the Restorative category of service, but what about reporting the provisional implant crown procedure?**

   CDT 2017 filled this procedure reporting gap by addition of **D6085 provisional implant crown** (a provisional implant crown can either abutment or implant supported). This procedure is similar to other provisional codes (e.g., **D2799 provisional crown**) in that there is neither a requirement that the provisional implant crown be used for a specific time period, nor prohibition on use if the final impression for the permanent implant crown has been taken. Keep in mind, an insurance carrier may not cover this procedure or make the code inclusive of the final prosthesis. Report D6085 for each affected tooth.

10. **My patient presents with a complete lower denture made 11 months ago at another dental office. She is unhappy with the fit and now realizes she should have had the implants her dentist recommended. Is there any way we can still use her existing denture after we place the implants and locator attachments?**

Yes, the existing denture can be used. This is a retrofitting procedure where the internal surface of the existing denture is modified to accommodate the retentive elements. The code is:

> **D5875 modification of removable prostheses following implant surgery**
> Attachment assemblies are reported using separate codes.

The locators and any relines are reported separately.

11. **An implant (D6010) I placed two years ago is failing and needs to be extracted due to peri-implantitis. Why is the insurance carrier asking me for a narrative? Does the carrier think I did something wrong?**

No. **D6100 implant removal** is a "by report" procedure code and a narrative must be submitted with the claim to describe the procedure. The narrative should include the location of the implant removed and the description of the procedure performed. It is also helpful to the carrier to say when the implant was initially placed, as well as to provide a radiographic image.

There may be other dental codes that you may use when you are removing the implant. The most likely would be a bone grafting code. The bone grafting dental code to use is the same that you use when extracting a tooth, which is D7953.

12. **I placed an abutment (D6056) and an abutment supported porcelain fused to metal crown (D6059). Six months later the patient presented with the implant crown in his hand. I took a radiographic image which showed no concerns with the implant fixture or abutment so I cemented the implant crown back in his mouth. Is there a code for this procedure?**

Yes, the code you would use is:

> **D6092 re-cement or re-bond implant/abutment supported crown**

13. **My patient comes in every three months for periodontal maintenance (D4910). She has all of her teeth with the exception of implants on teeth #2 and 4 which I placed one year ago and the restorative dentist has since placed the abutments and abutment supported crowns. She noticed bleeding around the implants after the implant crowns were placed so she came to my office to have them evaluated. I took a radiographic image and noticed that around both of her implants the gingival tissue was inflamed due to excess cement from the implant crown placement. However, there were no threads exposed and no bone loss present.**

    I need to scale and debride around the implants; should I use the code D4346?

    No. For scaling and debridement of the implants, use **D6081**. You would submit it twice – once for #2 and also for #4 since this is a per implant code.

    D6081 scaling and debridement in the presence of inflammation or mucositis of a single implant, including cleaning of the implant surfaces, without flap entry and closure

    This procedure is not performed in conjunction with D1110, D4910 or D4346.

14. **My patient had three implants placed last year by another dentist in another state and she is new to the area. Upon initial exam she complained that "all three implants are loose." Upon reviewing her medical history she is a chronic smoker and uncontrolled diabetic which is most likely why the implants failed. I will be removing the implants as well as placing bone graft material and a membrane.**

    I will use code D6100 implant removal, by report; does this code include the bone graft material and membrane?

    You are correct to use **D6100 implant removal, by report**. However this code does not include the bone graft or membrane. **D7953 bone replacement graft for ridge preservation-per site** is the proper code for the graft material, along with one of the following codes to report barrier membrane placement:

    D4266 guided tissue regeneration – resorbable barrier, per site

    or **D4267 guided tissue regeneration – non-resorbable barrier, per site (includes membrane removal)**

15. My patient has an implant on tooth #7 which was placed 4 years ago. The implant is well integrated with the bone and the patient is happy with the esthetics of the crown. However there is now slight recession present on the buccal and I plan on performing a connective tissue graft. But I can't find a code in the implant section. What code would I use?

The correct soft tissue graft codes are located in the Periodontics section and the code you choose depends on if you are performing an autogenous or non- autogenous connective tissue graft:

D4273 autogenous connective tissue graft procedure (including donor and recipient surgical sites) first tooth, implant or edentulous tooth position in graft

D4275 non-autogenous connective tissue graft (including recipient site and donor material) first tooth, implant, or edentulous tooth position in graft

16. D6010 surgical placement of an implant body does not include placement of a healing cap. The implant has osseointegrated and is ready to be uncovered. What code would be used for placement of a healing cap?

Surgical exposure of the implant is called "uncovering" or "second stage surgery" and is reported separately as **D6011**. The CDT definition of **D6011 second stage implant surgery** is "surgical access to an implant body for placement of a healing cap or to enable placement of an abutment." Note that some benefit plans consider this procedure to be inclusive under **D6010**.

17. Is an interim abutment the same as a healing cap?

No. An interim abutment D6051 is used while awaiting definitive treatment during a healing phase and is ultimately replaced by either **D6056 prefabricated abutment** or **D6057 custom fabricated abutment**. A healing cap is placed at the time of second stage surgery and just maintains an access opening to the implant body prior to the restorative phase of implant treatment.

18. What code reports blocking out an implant restorative access hole?

There was a request to add a code for this procedure in CDT 2018. However, the Code Maintenance Committee (CMC) did not accept the request for a separate CDT code as the committee considers blocking out an implant restorative access hole to be a component of the implant crown procedure.

However, if you block out an implant restorative access hole beyond the normal practice or if the patient loses the composite in the access hole of his implant crown, then submit as **D6199 unspecified implant procedure, by report** along with a detailed narrative.

19. Is there a code for an immediate implant placement?

There is no distinction in the surgical implant placement codes. They can be submitted whether the implant is placed at the time of tooth extraction or post extraction.

Summary

Coding for implants may appear challenging. However, it can be straightforward once you learn the basics. Some coding rules of thumb are in the following charts:

When the Final Prosthesis Is an Implant Crown or a Fixed Bridge

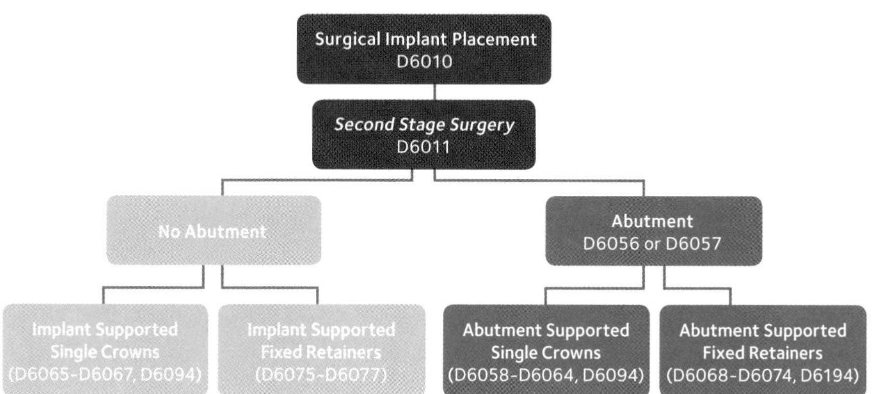

When the Final Prosthesis is a Removable or Fixed Implant Denture

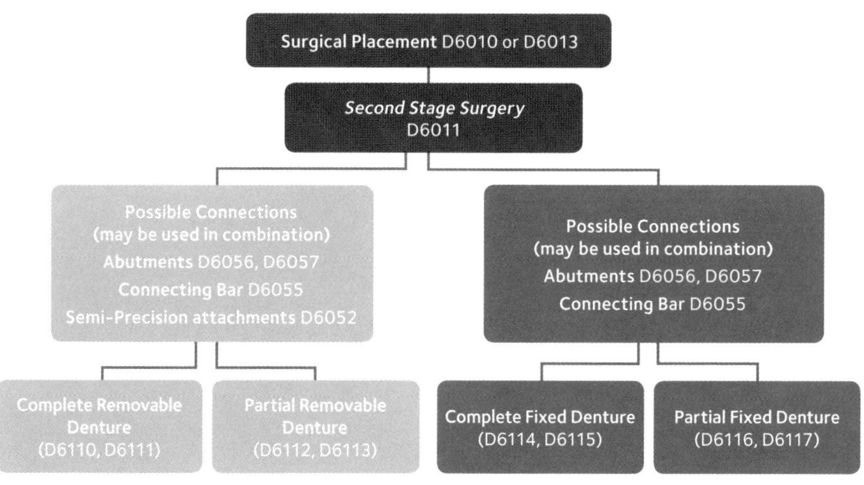

Reimbursement for surgical implant placement and restorations varies among dental benefit plans. Often when the surgical implant is not a benefit, the implant restorations are reimbursed as an alternative benefit. Even if a patients benefit plan does have implant coverage or has an implant rider, there still may be limitations and may not mean the plan includes benefits for implant maintenance related procedures. Pre-authorizing implants is highly recommended and may be a requirement of some patients' plans. A written estimate for the total cost of treatment – regardless of insurance coverage – should be presented, signed by the patient, and retained in the patient`s file.

Contributor Biography

Linda Vidone, D.M.D. is the Chief Clinical Officer/VP Clinical Management at Delta Dental of Massachusetts. She has 20 years of dental experience in clinical private practice, as dental school faculty, and in the dental benefits industry. Dr. Vidone, a board certified dental consultant, is a hands-on leader in the dental insurance industry, setting clinical policies and performing routine claim review while staying abreast of innovations in oral health care. She shares her unique knowledge of being on both sides of the claim form while lecturing nationwide on all aspects of dental benefits, dental coding, claim accuracy, utilization management and utilization review.

A graduate of Boston University School of Dental Medicine, Dr. Vidone holds a DMD and CAGS in General Dentistry and Periodontology. She is currently a member of the Delta Dental Plan Association Policy Committee. She also serves as Chair of the Certification Committee and is president of the American Association of Dental Consultants. She also maintains a private practice in periodontology in Brookline, Massachusetts.

Chapter 9.
D6200 – D6999 Prosthodontics, Fixed

By Teresa Duncan, M.S.

Introduction

Fixed prosthodontics replace missing teeth using fabricated materials that are cemented into onto existing natural teeth or roots. A dentist can choose from replacing missing teeth with an implant, fixed bridgework or removable partials and dentures. When treatment planning for fixed prosthodontics, it is important to remember that multiple appointments and procedures are usually required. Clinicians must take into account the patient's oral health habits along with existing restorations in order to determine if a fixed prosthetic is the best choice. Because many of the procedures can span over several appointments, it is advisable to inform the patient of the number of visits required.

Patients are often confused by the terminology used when discussing fixed prosthodontics. A treatment coordinator may be referring to a fixed partial denture between teeth #13 and 15, but the patient may not understand that this is the same as fixed bridgework. With implant and fixed restorations, it is helpful to have visual aids and even tangible examples on hand. Consider adding models, videos and images to your case presentation tools. Often the only time the patient has even seen a bridge or fixed partial denture is right before it is cemented into his or her mouth.

From the beginning, your team should use the same language when discussing the components of fixed prosthodontics. They should also keep in mind that although most fixed prosthodontics are cemented permanently there can be situations in which the practitioner will choose to do so temporarily.

Key Definitions and Concepts

Retainer: For years the retainer was referred to as the "abutment" but as implant usage and coding has evolved, it has shifted away from that. A retainer acts as a stabilizer for the prosthodontic.

Abutment: When discussing fixed prosthodontics, the abutment is the part of the tooth upon which the retainer will seat. There may be times when additional buildup material is needed for an ideal restoration.

Pontic: An artificial tooth created to take the place of a missing tooth. It will be attached to retainers. There is no supporting tooth or root below it. It may rest against but is not meant to be supported by the soft tissue. As bone resorbs, the soft tissue may pull away from the pontic.

Connector: The part that unifies the pontic and the retainer.

Fixed Partial Denture: A laboratory fabricated prosthetic that replaces missing teeth or empty tooth spaces. It is meant to stabilize the bite and maintain arch integrity. This means that it prevents teeth from shifting and changing the patient's bite which can lead to future required treatment. Also referred to as fixed bridgework or a bridge.

Cantilever Bridge: A fixed partial denture (bridge) in which a stabilizing retainer is not present on one end.

Changes to This Category

There are no changes to this category in CDT 2019 (nor were there any in CDT 2018 or 2017).

Diagnosis Codes – ICD-10-CM

The CDT to ICD tables in Appendix 1 provide appropriate guidance on linkages between "Prosthodontics, fixed" procedure codes and diagnosis codes.

Note: Fixed prosthodontics services are typically not reimbursable under medical plans. If it is necessary to cross-code these services, then the diagnosis for tooth loss, oral condition or any systemic conditions should be referenced.

CODING SCENARIO #1

Cantilever Bridge

A patient presents with tooth #27 missing and the dentist learned that this tooth has been missing for under a year. The dentist also observed that teeth #26 and 28 appeared to be in good condition. Upon further evaluation, the dentist determined that tooth #26 would not provide enough retention for a Maryland bridge and was reluctant to incorporate a virgin tooth in the prosthetic.

The patient was presented the information regarding Maryland bridge replacement and cantilever bridge replacement, with the doctor recommending a cantilever bridge off tooth #28 to preserve #26's tooth structure. The patient reviewed the informed consent and opted for the cantilever bridge procedure.

What codes are used to document and report this procedure?

Tooth #28 is a retainer and the applicable code is:

D6750 retainer crown - porcelain fused to high noble metal

Note: Retainers are differentiated by their material. Examples include:

- D6751 retainer crown – porcelain fused to predominantly base metal
- D6752 retainer crown – porcelain fused to noble metal
- D6780 retainer crown – 3/4 cast high noble metal

(Refer to CDT 2019 for the full list of applicable codes based on the prosthetic's material.)

The pontic code for a "cantilever" bridge are the same as a conventional bridge, which for tooth #27 would be:

D6240 pontic – porcelain fused to high noble metal

As with the retainers, pontics may be made of different material. Always refer to CDT 2019 to use the appropriate code.

CODING SCENARIO #2

A Maryland Bridge

A patient suffered an accident that damaged the dentition as follows:

- Two teeth were lost – #23 and #24
- One tooth was broken – #26

The doctor determined that #26 could not be restored and required extraction.

The initial treatment plan involved implants, which the patient declined due to cost. An alternative treatment plan was accepted. This alternative involved a Maryland bridge as this would preserve the remaining teeth and retain the option of implant in the future. The Maryland bridge consisted of a resin bonded porcelain-fused-to-metal (noble) bridge from teeth #22 to #27 with #25 acting as a pier.

What codes are used to document and report this procedure?

Teeth #22, 25 and 27 become retainers and the applicable code for each is:

D6545 retainer – cast metal for resin bonded fixed prosthesis

The pontic codes for a Maryland bridge are the same as a conventional bridge, which for teeth #23, 24, and 26 is (reported for each):

D6242 pontic – porcelain fused to noble metal

Note: Resin bonded bridge retainers (often referred to as wings) are differentiated by their material:

- All cast metal or porcelain fused to metal bridges would utilize the **D6545** code noted above.
- The porcelain/ceramic retainer code (**D6548**) could only be used with a porcelain/ceramic pontic.
- Should the retainer be fabricated out of resin/composite, the applicable CDT code is **D6549 resin retainer – for resin bonded fixed prosthesis**.

CODING SCENARIO #3

Three-Unit Fixed Partial Denture (Bridge) for Teeth #12-14 with Buildup on Molar Tooth

The patient presented with an existing fixed partial denture that needed to be replaced, and the dentist also determined that a gingivectomy would be necessary. The patient was presented the treatment plan and gave informed consent. Upon removal of the existing prosthetic the treating dentist decided that a buildup was needed to properly restore the molar tooth.

Removal of the existing decay necessitated the addition of buildup material, and the dentist informed the patient of the change in treatment.

How would you code this scenario's treatment plan?

The initial treatment plan was for a replacement fixed partial denture involving teeth #12-14 and documented with the following codes:

#12 **D4212 gingivectomy or gingivoplasty to allow access for restorative procedure, per tooth**

#12 **D6752 retainer crown – porcelain fused to noble metal**

#13 **D6242 pontic – porcelain fused to noble metal**

#14 **D6752 retainer crown – porcelain fused to noble metal**

A flap of gingiva was prohibiting proper preparation of the tooth for the retainer crown so D4212 was appropriate in this situation. The next decision was which material to use for the fixed partial denture. The doctor decided to use porcelain fused to noble metal based on soft tissue and material selection criteria.

When the treatment plan changed to include the buildup the code below was added:

#14 **D2950 core buildup, including any pins when required**

It is important to note that this code is located in the Restorative section of the CDT manual.

CODING SCENARIO #4

Fractured Tooth and Infection

A patient presents with painful and fractured tooth #5. The doctor took a radiograph that imaged the entire tooth as part of the focused oral evaluation. A two-phase treatment plan was presented and accepted. Descriptions of each phase, and applicable coding, follow.

How would you code each phase in this scenario?

First Phase

- Evaluation and diagnosis
- Extraction of #5 – no need to remove bone
- Impression of the extraction area and adjacent hard and soft tissues
- Creation and placement of a temporary fixed partial denture for healing and space maintenance

Codes for first phase procedures:

	D0140	**limited oral evaluation – problem focused**
	D0220	**intraoral – periapical first radiographic image**
#4	**D6793**	**provisional retainer crown – further treatment or completion of diagnosis necessary prior to final impression**
#5	**D7140**	**extraction, erupted tooth or exposed root (elevation and/or forceps removal)**
#5	**D6253**	**provisional pontic – further treatment or completion of diagnosis necessary prior to final impression**
#6	**D6793**	**provisional retainer crown – further treatment or completion of diagnosis necessary prior to final impression**

Second Phase

- Place permanent fixed partial denture

Codes for second phase procedures:

#4	**D6740**	**retainer crown – porcelain/ceramic**
#5	**D6245**	**pontic – porcelain/ceramic**
#6	**D6740**	**retainer crown – porcelain/ceramic**

CODING SCENARIO #5

Existing Bridge Has Come Loose

A patient presents for a limited evaluation with bridge in hand. The bridge spanned teeth #13-15. Two periapical radiographs were taken and reviewed to assess health and stability of the teeth. An existing full set of radiographs had been taken within the last year. It was determined that no new caries was present and that the bridge could be re-cemented. The patient accepted this recommendation. After cleaning of the existing restoration, the bridge was re-cemented and post-care instructions were given.

How would you code this scenario?

The patient presented for an evaluation and had radiographs taken and reviewed. The bridge was then re-cemented.

D0140 limited oral evaluation – problem focused

D0220 intraoral – periapical first radiographic image

D0230 intraoral – each additional radiographic image

D6930 re-cement or re-bond fixed partial denture

Coding Q&A

1. **Should I present a treatment plan for an implant if my recommendation is to place a fixed partial denture?**

   Yes, you should always present all available options to the patient. The patient must be aware of all the options available to restore their oral condition. However, you can present a recommended treatment. Patients rely on our candid advice when making their dental decisions.

2. **What if a child presents for treatment and needs more than a space maintainer? Can I recommend a purely aesthetic fixed partial denture to maintain that tooth space?**

   Code **D6985 pediatric partial denture, fixed** is perfect for this scenario. It should be noted that the code encompasses all parts for this type of fixed partial denture. There is no separate reporting of retainers or pontics.

3. **We have had to temporarily cement fixed bridgework. Is there a separate code for that?**

   Sometimes a fixed partial denture is temporarily cemented so that the clinician can observe the oral condition for a time period. If the fixed partial denture is intended to be the permanent restoration, then there is not a separate code. You are simply delaying the permanent delivery. You may want to use code **D6999 unspecified fixed prosthodontic procedure, by report** to request reimbursement. This will require a narrative and supporting images.

4. **Our patient presented with a multi-unit bridge that had come out. It is a large bridge with five pontics and five retainers. Can we charge the re-cement fee for multiple teeth?**

   Existing code **D6930 re-cement or re-bond fixed partial denture** is per prosthetic. The number of units is not a factor.

5. **I'd like to place a post and core buildup in a tooth that previously had endodontic therapy. This tooth will serve as an abutment in a bridge. Is the code found in this section or in Endodontics?**

   The post and core procedure codes are actually found in the CDT Code's Restorative category of service.

   D2952 post and core in addition to crown, indirectly fabricated

   D2954 prefabricated post and core in addition to crown

   There is no post and core buildup code that is specific to only crowns or only fixed partial dentures.

6. **I would like to place a temporary bridge while a site is healing. We are planning to treat adjacent teeth but would like to preserve the tooth space in the meantime. What code should I use?**

   You are referring to a provisional fixed partial denture which includes codes D6973 for the provisional retainer and D6253 for the provisional pontic.

7. **I plan to use a precision attachment. Do I bill for the male and female component separately?**

   The precision attachment code D6950 includes both the male and female part, and should be billed per tooth.

Summary

The selection of a fixed prosthodontics code should be made with the following items in mind:

1. Material used in restoration.
2. Is it to replace a missing tooth or tooth space?
3. Is the end result meant to be part of a permanent placement?
4. Diagnostic procedures are separate from fixed prosthodontic codes.
5. Any soft tissue preparation is separate from the fixed prosthodontic code.

In some situations, a fixed prosthetic is part of an implant case. Specifically, the pontic codes for a fixed partial denture that is supported by implants are found in the fixed prosthodontic section. There are no pontic codes that are specific to implant restoration cases.

If you cannot find an appropriate code for your procedure, then use:

D6999 unspecified fixed prosthodontic procedure, by report

When using a "by report" code remember to include a diagnosis, description of procedure and prognosis. Include any supporting documentation such as radiographs and intraoral images.

Contributor Biography

Teresa Duncan, M.S. is the president of Odyssey Management, Inc. Her company provides courses in the areas of insurance and revenue administration. She may be reached via her website *www.OdysseyMgmt.com*. Her website contains many management and insurance articles, as well as complimentary webinars.

Chapter 10. D7000 – D7999 Oral and Maxillofacial Surgery

By James Mercer, D.D.S.

Introduction

Oral and maxillofacial surgery is a broad area. It encompasses not only the discipline of oral surgery, but also that of implant services, radiologic imaging, trauma, facial cosmetic procedures and anesthesia services. Some of the procedures are medical in nature and need to be submitted to medical carriers along with ICD-10-CM codes. However, there are still many procedures which are purely dental in nature.

Key Definitions and Concepts

Autogenous Graft: A graft that is taken from one part of a patient's body and transferred to another.

Anesthesia Definitions: A patient's level of consciousness is determined by the anesthesia provider's documentation of a patient's level of consciousness and is not dependent upon the route of administration of anesthesia.

Deep Sedation: A drug-induced depression of consciousness during which patients cannot be easily aroused but respond purposefully following repeated or painful stimulation. The ability to independently maintain ventilator function may be impaired. Patients may require assistance in maintaining a patent airway. Cardiovascular function is usually maintained.

General Anesthesia: A drug-induced loss of consciousness during which patients are not arousable. The ability to maintain ventilator function is often impaired. Cardiovascular function may be impaired.

Minimal Sedation: A minimally depressed level of consciousness that retains the patient's ability to independently and continuously maintain an airway and respond normally to tactile stimulation and verbal command. Ventilatory and cardiovascular functions are unaffected.

Moderate Sedation: A drug-induced depression of consciousness during which patients respond purposefully to verbal commands either alone or accompanied by light tactile stimulation. Spontaneous ventilation is adequate. Cardiovascular function is usually maintained.

Anxiolysis: The diminution or elimination of anxiety.

Provisional: Formed or preformed for temporary purposes or used over a limited period.

Soft Tissue Impacted Tooth: Occlusal surface of the tooth is covered by soft tissue.

Partial Bone Impacted Tooth: Part of the crown is covered by bone.

Full Bone Impacted Tooth: Most or all of the crown is covered by bone.

Changes to This Category

There was one change to this category of service in CDT 2019:

D7283 placement of device to facilitate eruption of impacted tooth
Placement of an ~~orthodontic bracket, band or other device~~ attachment on an unerupted tooth, after its exposure, to aid in its eruption. Report the surgical exposure separately using D7280.

The rational to eliminate the phrase "orthodontic bracket, band or other device" and use the word "attachment" demonstrates that this procedure can be done for purposes other than orthodontics. On many occasions, insurance companies see "orthodontic" in the descriptor (or even in the nomenclature) and deduct the claim payment from the orthodontic coverage although no orthodontic treatment was performed.

An example where this code would apply is an attachment which is placed after surgical exposure of a mesially impacted permanent first molar that is trapped by the deciduous second molar. The attachment is designed to "unlock" the permanent first molar and allow normal eruption. No orthodontics are being done and may never be done to achieve eruption.

Diagnosis Codes – ICD-10-CM

The CDT to ICD tables in Appendix 1 provide appropriate guidance on linkages between often used Oral and Maxillofacial Surgery procedure codes and diagnosis codes. There are, in addition, ICD-10-CM codes not in these tables that may be applicable in some situations, or for procedures not listed.

F41.9 anxiety disorder, unspecified
K08.12 complete loss of teeth due to periodontal diseases
K08.13 complete loss of teeth due to caries
K08.20 unspecified atrophy of edentulous alveolar ridge
K08.21 minimal atrophy of the mandible
K08.22 moderate atrophy of the mandible
K08.23 minimal atrophy of the mandible
K08.24 minimal atrophy of the maxilla
K08.25 moderate atrophy of the maxilla
K08.26 severe atrophy of the maxilla
K11.5 sialolithiasis
K11.6 mucocele of salivary gland
K12.0 recurrent oral aphthae
M26.60 temporomandibular joint disorder, unspecified

CODING SCENARIO #1

Connective Tissue Grafts – Autogenous and Non-autogenous

A 55-year-old male who is a patient of record presented to an oral surgeon's office six years after placement of two separate implants for tooth #s 12 and 13. Exam revealed loss of 3 mm of attached gingiva on the buccal aspect of the implants. X-rays revealed minimal bone loss on the implants. There was one thread on each implant exposed. Along with debridement of the area, the treatment plan consisted of placing a connective tissue graft on the buccal of both implants.

How would you code for the autogenous grafts?

D4273 autogenous connective tissue graft procedure (including donor and recipient surgical sites) first tooth, implant or edentulous tooth position in graft

D4283 autogenous connective tissue graft procedure (including donor and recipient surgical sites) – each additional contiguous implant in same graft site

Note: D4273 is the code used when the procedure involves two surgical sites, donor and recipient. The recipient site has a split thickness incision and the connective tissue is from a separate donor site leaving an epithelized flap for closure. D4283 is used to code for additional sites adjacent to the first site.

If using a non-autogenous connective graft, the procedures are coded as follows:

D4275 non-autogenous connective tissue graft (including recipient site and donor material) first tooth, implant or edentulous tooth position in graft

D4285 non-autogenous connective tissue graft procedure (including recipient surgical site and donor material) – each additional contiguous tooth, implant and edentulous tooth position in the same graft site

CODING SCENARIO #2

Harvesting Bone and Hard Tissue Grafting

Two years following an ATV accident, the patient was still dealing with the after effects of the comminuted fracture of his anterior maxilla. A traumatic defect and oro-nasal fistula, not much different from a congenital alveolar cleft, still existed.

The patient's oral surgeon recommended closure of the fistula and reconstruction of the bony deficit prior to prosthetic reconstruction. The doctor planned to do this as an in office procedure utilizing an autogenous bone graft from the tibia.

What codes would be used to document these procedures?

Two codes would be used to document the planned services to be delivered in the doctor's office:

D7955 **repair of maxillofacial soft tissue and/or hard tissue defect**
Reconstruction of surgical, traumatic, or congenital defects of the facial bones, including the mandible, may utilize graft materials in conjunction with soft tissue procedures to repair and restore the facial bones to form and function. This does not include obtaining the graft.

D7295 **harvest of bone for use in autogenous grafting procedure**
Reported in addition to those autogenous graft placement procedures that do not include harvesting of bone.

Note: The harvesting code **D7295** was added in CDT 2011. This addition provides a means to report the separate procedure of obtaining osseous material for the purpose of grafting to a distant site. It enables documentation of the harvesting procedure when the grafting procedure (e.g., **D4263**; **D7953**; **D7955**) does not include obtaining bone to be grafted.

CODING SCENARIO #3

Implant Placement with Inadequate Bone Volume

A 36 year-old female patient presents for placement of an implant in the mandibular right posterior. Tooth #30 had been extracted two years ago. There is inadequate bone volume in the site where the implant will be placed and ridge augmentation is required.

How do you code for the graft?

D7950 osseous, periosteal, or cartilage graft of the mandible or maxilla – autogenous or nonautogenous, by report
This procedure is for ridge augmentation or reconstruction to increase height, width and/or volume of residual alveolar ridge. It includes obtaining graft material. Placement of a barrier membrane, if used, should be reported separately.

How do you code for the barrier membrane if used?

D4266 guided tissue regeneration – resorbable barrier, per site

or **D4267 guided tissue regeneration – non-resorbable barrier, per site (includes membrane removal)**

CODING SCENARIO #4

Autogenous Bone Graft

A 45-year-old male presents for extraction of non-restorable tooth #5 and placement of an implant at a later date. An autogenous bone graft is placed with a membrane at the time of extraction to increase the bone volume and preserve ridge integrity at the future implant site.

After coding for the extraction, how do you code for the graft and membrane portion of the procedure?

D7953 bone replacement graft for ridge preservation – per site
Graft is placed in an extraction site or implant removal site at the time of the extraction or removal to preserve ridge integrity (e.g., clinically indicated in preparation for implant reconstruction or where alveolar contour is critical to planned prosthetic reconstruction). Does not include obtaining graft material. Membrane, if used should be reported separately.

D7295 harvest of bone for use in autogenous grafting procedure
Reported in addition to those autogenous graft placement procedures that do not include harvesting of bone.

D4266 guided tissue regeneration – resorbable barrier, per site

or **D4267 guided tissue regeneration – non-resorbable barrier, per site (includes membrane removal)**

How would you code for this procedure if the implant is placed at the same time of the extraction and the graft?

D6010 surgical placement of implant body: endosteal implant

D6104 bone graft at time of implant placement
Placement of a barrier membrane, or biologic materials to aid in osseous regeneration are reported separately.

What code would also be reported if a barrier membrane were placed?

D4266 guided tissue regeneration – resorbable barrier, per site

or **D4267 guided tissue regeneration – non-resorbable barrier, per site (includes membrane removal)**

CODING SCENARIO #5

Diagnostic Work-Up – New Patient

An 18-year-old female patient presented to an oral surgeon, referred from an orthodontist for evaluation of her mandibular retrognathia. After examination, it was noted that she had a full adult dentition in good repair with a 6 mm retrognathic mandible. In order to complete the diagnostic work-up, the surgeon obtained a panoramic image, a cephalometric radiograph, models and a bite registration and extra-oral photographs.

How would you code for this visit?

D0150 comprehensive oral exam – new or established patient

The comprehensive exam is delivered because this is a new patient of record and required a thorough evaluation of both intra-oral and extra-oral hard and soft tissues. It also involves the recording of the patient's dental and medical history.

D0330 panoramic radiographic image

D0340 2D cephalometric radiographic image – acquisition, measurement and analysis

The cephalometric image is made using a cephalostat to standardize anatomic positioning and is reproducible.

D0350 2D oral/facial photographic image obtained intra-orally or extra-orally

CODING SCENARIO #6

Possible Orbital Fracture

A 23-year-old male presents to the office after being punched in the face the night before. He has severe periorbital swelling of the left eye. The surgeon is unable to perform an adequate clinical exam and does not have a CBCT in the office. But she does have a cephalometric x-ray machine capable of taking a flat plate extra-oral film. She takes a Waters view film to rule-out an orbital fracture.

How do you code for this diagnostic imaging procedure?

D0250 extra-oral – 2D projection radiographic image created using a stationary radiation source, and detector

D0250 covers a class of images which can be obtained utilizing a flat plate radiographic image to view aspects of the skull and facial bones when a CBCT scan is not available.

CODING SCENARIO #7

Extraction of Full Bony Impacted Teeth

A 20-year-old male presents to the oral surgeon's office for extraction of full bony impacted teeth #1, 16, 17 and 32. The procedure was performed utilizing deep IV sedation. The procedure lasted 53 minutes.

How would you code for the deep sedation anesthesia procedure?

D9222 deep sedation/general anesthesia – first 15 minutes

D9223 deep sedation/general anesthesia – each subsequent 15 minute increment

Report D9222 once for minutes one through 15, and D9223 three times for the additional 38 minutes (16 through 53). D9223 documents each additional full or partial 15-minute increment.

What code would be reported if 53 minutes of moderate IV sedation were appropriate?

D9239 intravenous moderate (conscious) sedation/analgesia – first 15 minutes

D9243 intravenous moderate (conscious) sedation/analgesia – each subsequent 15 minute increment

Procedure code D9239 would be reported once and D9243 three times on the claim.

What code would be reported if the extraction procedure could be performed with non-IV conscious sedation?

D9248 non-intravenous conscious sedation

This procedure would be reported once as it is not time-based.

CODING SCENARIO #8

Orthognathic Surgery Planning

An oral and maxillofacial surgery office recently installed a cone beam radiography machine. It was used to treatment plan some anticipated orthognathic surgery for a patient. Following image capture, several axial and lateral views were constructed to plan the surgery. A panoramic view was also produced to send to the patient's orthodontist.

After consultation with the orthodontist, the surgeon constructed a 3D virtual model, which they viewed together on the computer, to properly locate a temporary implant to anchor the orthodontic appliance. The virtual model could be manipulated on the screen to allow them to visualize other anatomical structures in the area and their relationship to the teeth to determine the ideal location to place the implant.

A transmucosal endosseous implant was placed as a temporary fixation device for the patient's braces. The temporary implant will be removed when orthodontic treatment is completed.

How could you code for procedures delivered during the initial treatment planning visit (includes initial scan, coronal and sagittal views, and panoramic view)?

D0367 cone beam CT capture and interpretation with field of view of both jaws; with or without cranium

This code was added effective January 1, 2013 specifically to report procedures related to cone beam imaging technology. It replaces the separate cone beam data capture (**D0360**) and two-dimension reconstruction (**D0362**) codes. The image capture includes two-dimensional sectional (tomographic) views from the axial (coronal or frontal) and lateral (sagittal) planes, as well as the panoramic view.

How could you code the subsequent consultation procedure (3D virtual model)?

D0393 treatment simulation using 3D image volume

The 3D virtual model is a three-dimensional image reconstructed from data acquired during the treatment planning visit.

How could you code the temporary implant placement procedure that required a surgical flap?

D7293 placement of temporary anchorage device requiring flap; includes device removal

Temporary implants also represent a new kind of technology for which codes were added effective January 1, 2007. The correct code to use for this type of implant depends upon whether it will be used for fixation or an interim restoration. In this case, the implant is being used as a fixation device for orthodontics, so the correct code comes from the CDT Code's Oral and Maxillofacial Surgery category.

Note: If the temporary implant does not require a surgical flap, the correct code would be **D7294 placement of temporary anchorage device without flap; includes device removal**.

CODING SCENARIO #9

Treating a Traumatic Wound a Mouthguard Could Have Prevented

An eight-year-old patient arrived at the oral and maxillofacial surgeon's office literally screaming. The doctor understood why when he saw the patient who was injured during a baseball game. A headfirst slide had resulted in a lower lip full of gravel and a chin raspberry in the making.

An intramuscular injection of 40mg of ketamine provided a reasonable amount of sedation and allowed sufficient time to completely debride the wound, followed by placing sutures in the cut in the patient's lip. No teeth were broken. The doctor recommended a mouthguard for protection.

What codes would be used to document and report procedures delivered during this visit?

The CDT Code for a parenteral sedative is:

D9248 non-intravenous conscious sedation

Note: Effective January 1, 2007, **D9610 therapeutic drug injection, by report** was revised to exclude the reporting of sedative agents.

There is not a code for traumatic wound debridement, but **D7999 unspecified oral surgery procedure, by report** could be used for that procedure.

Suture placement is reported with a code based on the size of the wound:

D7910 suture of recent small wounds up to 5cm

The code to use when making a mouthguard:

D9941 fabrication of athletic mouthguard

CODING SCENARIO #10

Coronectomy

An oral and maxillofacial surgeon completed consultations with two patients, both of whom faced similar complications.

Patient 1

A 38-year-old male presents with chronic pericoronitis associated with a deep mesio-angular impaction of tooth #32. There is gingival inflammation and substantial bone loss surrounding the crown. The root of the tooth extends well past the inferior alveolar nerve canal and it is the dentist's opinion that removal of the entire tooth is a substantial risk to the nerve.

Patient 2

A 19-year-old female presents for evaluation and treatment of a dentigerous cyst, associated with an impacted supernumerary tooth in the area of #20, displaced inferiorly and is encroaching on the left mental foramen. After evaluation and examination, the dentist determines that total removal of the supernumerary tooth risks injury to the inferior alveolar nerve.

What procedure codes would be used to document the services delivered today, and planned for a future date?

Each patient's record would have the same procedure codes.

For today's consultation:

D9310 consultation – diagnostic service provided by dentist or physician other than requesting dentist or physician

For the planned procedure:

D7251 coronectomy – intentional partial tooth removal

Note: **D7251** was added to the Code on Dental Procedures and Nomenclature effective January 1, 2011. Its addition enables documentation of intentional partial tooth removal that is performed when a neurovascular complication is likely if the entire impacted tooth is removed. The procedure avoids complications involving the inferior alveolar nerve and the lingual nerve.

CODING SCENARIO #11

Oroantral Fistula

A 23-year-old male is referred to the oral surgeon for evaluation of a partial boney impacted tooth #1. A clinical exam reveals pain on palpation. A panoramic image shows that the roots are in close proximity to the sinus and that there is no cystic lesion present. The procedure for the extraction of #1 is reviewed including risks and alternate treatments. The patient elects to have the tooth removed utilizing general anesthesia.

The patient returns for the surgery. After extracting the tooth, a large oroantral opening is noted and a mucoperiosteal flap is elevated with a buccal releasing incision to obtain primary closure. The procedure takes 20 minutes and the patient heals without incident.

How do you code for procedures related to the surgery encounter?

D7230 removal of impacted tooth – partially bony
Part of crown covered by bone; requires mucoperiosteal flap elevation and bone removal.

D7261 primary closure of a sinus perforation
Subsequent to surgical removal of tooth, exposure of sinus requiring repair, or immediate closure of oroantral or oronasal communication in absence of fistulous tract.

D9222 deep sedation/general anesthesia – first 15 minutes

D9223 deep sedation/general anesthesia – each subsequent 15 minute increment

If during the extraction there was no oroantral opening but the patient returned a few weeks later with an oroantral opening with a fistulous tract but no signs of infection, and the oroantral opening was closed at this subsequent visit with a primary closure, what would be the correct code for the closure procedure?

D7260 oroantral fistula closure
Excision of fistulous tract between maxillary sinus and oral cavity and closure by advancement flap.

CODING SCENARIO #12

TMD Therapy

You have been treating a 32-year-old female who previously presented with complaints of several years of headaches, facial pain and "popping" in her left TM joint with occasional locking. Her treatment plan includes but is not limited to a splint for her temporomandibular joint dysfunction and in-office physical therapy.

How do you code for the device and physical therapy?

D7880 occlusal orthotic device, by report
Presently includes splints provided for the treatment of temporomandibular joint dysfunction.

D9130 temporomandibular joint dysfunction – non-invasive physical therapies
Therapy including but not limited to massage, diathermy, ultrasound, or cold application to provide relief from muscle spasms, inflammation or pain, intending to improve freedom of motion and joint function. This should be reported on a per session basis.

You feel an MRI is needed to further evaluate the soft tissue of the joint. The mandible needs to be in a specific position at the time of the MRI and a device is used to position the mandible for the MRI.

How do you code for the device?

If the occlusal orthotic device is used that is also being used in her ongoing treatment, then no additional code is needed. If you construct an additional device to position the jaw for the MRI, then you may use:

D7899 unspecified TMD therapy, by report
Used for procedure that is not adequately described by a code. Describe procedure.

CODING SCENARIO #13

Hyperplastic Tissue Excision

A 77-year-old male presents with ill-fitting dentures and requests new dentures. You determine that prior to constructing new dentures, he will require excision of some excess tissue in the maxilla related to irritation from his current dentures.

How would you code for the excision in the maxilla using a laser vs. excision using a scalpel?

The codes are procedure based rather than instrument based. Therefore the same code is used for either instrumentation.

D7970 excision of hyperplastic tissue – per arch

CODING SCENARIO #14

Non-opioid Post-operative Pain Management

A 17-year-old female is referred for extraction of painful impacted teeth # 1, 16, 17, and 32. During the consultation, the patient's mother expresses concern about her daughter receiving opioids as part of the post-operative pain management protocol. To address this concern, following the manufacturer's instructions, the surgeon plans to infiltrate bupivacaine liposome injectable suspension at the surgical sites at the end of the procedure.

How would you code for the bupivacaine liposome injectable suspension?

D9613 infiltration of sustained release therapeutic drug – single or multiple sites

Infiltration of a sustained release pharmacologic agent for long acting surgical site pain control. Not for local anesthesia purposes.

Coding Q&A

1. A patient presents to the office for a follow up treatment for bruxing and an adjustment was made to his occlusal guard. What is the correct code?

   D9943 occlusal guard adjustment

2. An immediate implant and a provisional crown was placed in the #8 position. What is the proper code for the crown?

   D6085 provisional implant crown

3. A 75-year-old male with severe cardiac disease, including a history of aortic valve replacement, presents to the office for evaluation of his remaining dentition for extraction. The surgeon gives the patient antibiotics to be taken at home one hour prior to the scheduled appointment for his extractions. Due to the severity of his cardiac condition, the surgeon contacted the patient's cardiologist to discuss the planned procedure.

   How do you code for the medication and the phone consultation with the cardiologist?

   D9630 drugs or medicaments dispensed in the office for home use

   D9311 consultation with a medical health care professional

4. A patient needed an extraction, and it turned into a very difficult procedure. The doctor removed most of the tooth, but was unable to remove the entire root and the patient was referred to an oral surgeon immediately. Is there a code for a partial extraction?

   There are no partial extraction codes available. To report this procedure, use code **D7999 unspecified oral surgery procedure, by report**.

5. I removed a portion of the patient's fractured tooth, but not the entire tooth, to provide immediate relief of pain. How should I report this procedure?

   There is no code that specifically refers to removal of a portion of a fractured tooth to relieve pain. When there is no procedure code whose nomenclature and descriptor reflect the service provided, an "unspecified...procedure, by report" code may be considered (e.g., D7999 unspecified oral surgery procedure, by report).

6. **I am an oral surgeon and extracted a fully erupted tooth. My extractions are usually documented with CDT code D7210. For this patient, however, there was no need for any of the surgical actions listed in this code's nomenclature and descriptor. Is D7210 appropriate to document the service, or should I consider D7140?**

   Selection of the appropriate code comes through consideration of the full CDT Code entry, as follows:

   D7140 extraction, erupted tooth or exposed root (elevation and/or forceps removal)
   Includes routine removal of tooth structure, minor smoothing of socket bone, and closure, as necessary.

   D7210 extraction of erupted tooth requiring removal of bone and/or sectioning of tooth, and including elevation of mucoperiosteal flap if indicated
   Includes related cutting of gingiva and bone, removal of tooth structure, minor smoothing of socket bone and closure.

   As you did not perform any of the actions listed in the **D7210** nomenclature, D7140 is the only applicable CDT code to document and report the service.

7. **According to its descriptor code, "D7241 removal of impacted tooth - completely bony with unusual surgical complications" can be used for a completely impacted tooth with an "aberrant tooth position." Would a completely impacted wisdom tooth that is radiographically very close to the mandibular nerve justify use of this procedure code?**

   Perhaps. The dentist serving the patient is in the best position to determine whether the observed clinical condition of the patient's dentition and the procedure provided matches a dental procedure code (e.g., D7241). Radiographic images may not provide enough visual information to determine the extent of bony coverage, aberrant tooth position or other unusual circumstances.

   Should a dentist determine that a specific code does not adequately apply to the service rendered, we recommend that the service be reported using an "unspecified procedure, by report" code (e.g., D7999 unspecified oral surgery procedure, by report).

8. **Which soft tissue biopsy code should I use?**

There are three codes for soft tissue biopsies, differentiated by the depth and structural integrity of the tissue sample.

D7286 incisional biopsy of oral tissue – soft tissue
For partial removal of an architecturally intact specimen only. This procedure is not used at the same time as codes for apicoectomy/periradicular curettage. This procedure does not entail an excision.

D7287 exfoliative cytological sample collection
For collection of non-transepithelial cytology sample via mild scraping of the oral mucosa.

D7288 brush biopsy – transepithelial sample collection
For collection of oral disaggregated transepithelial cells via rotational brushing of the oral mucosa.

Code **D7286** would be used for incisional tissue samples that maintain the original structure. Codes **D7287** and **D7288** are used for cell sampling biopsies that do not maintain tissue architecture.

9. **What is the appropriate code for reporting a supra-crestal fiberotomy?**

The available procedure code for reporting a supra-crestal fiberotomy is **D7291 transseptal fiberotomy, by report**.

10. **What is a fibroma and how would removal be reported?**

A fibroma is a benign tumor composed of fibrous or connective tissue, and the available procedure codes are:

D7410 excision of benign lesion up to 1.25 cm

D7411 excision of benign lesion greater than 1.25 cm

11. **How do I code removal of mandibular tori?**

If the bony elevations are located lingually **D7473 removal of torus mandibularis** may be reported by quadrant.

12. What is a torus/exostosis and how would removal be reported?

A torus/exostosis is a benign overgrowth of bone forming an elevation or protuberance of bone. They can form in the patient's palate, lingual or lateral aspect of the maxilla or mandible.

Available procedure codes may include:

D7471 removal of lateral exostosis (maxilla or mandible)

D7472 removal of torus palatinus

D7473 removal of torus mandibularis

13. What is the difference between the procedures reported with the following three CDT codes?

D4263 bone replacement graft – retained natural tooth first site in quadrant

Report when the bone graft is performed to stimulate periodontal regeneration when the disease process has led to a deformity of the bone around an existing tooth.

D7950 osseous, periosteal, or cartilage graft of the mandible or maxilla – autogenous or nonautogenous, by report

Report when the graft is used for augmentation or reconstruction of an edentulous area of a ridge.

D7953 bone replacement graft for ridge preservation – per site

Report when the bone graft is placed in an extraction site at the time of the extraction to preserve ridge integrity.

14. How do I code the use of collagen wound dressing products that promote hemostasis (blood clotting)?

There is no procedure code for collagen wound dressing products. Use of collagen may be a component of a procedure such as "D9930 treatment of complications (post-surgical) – unusual circumstances, by report." In other circumstances, depending on the primary procedure performed, code "D7999 unspecified oral surgery procedure, by report" or "D4999 unspecified periodontal procedure, by report" may be reported.

15. How can I report a sinus lift procedure?

There are two codes available for different approaches:

D7951 sinus augmentation with bone or bone substitutes via a lateral open approach

D7952 sinus augmentation via a vertical approach

16. What is an operculectomy, and how would it be coded?

In dentistry, an operculum is a small flap of tissue surrounding or partially covering the back molars and "ectomy" is a suffix referring to the removal of something. Therefore, an operculectomy is the surgical removal of a flap of tissue surrounding a partially erupted or impacted tooth.

The available procedure code is:

D7971 excision of pericoronal gingiva
Removal of inflammatory or hypertrophied tissues surrounding partially erupted/impacted teeth.

17. The dentist performed a frenectomy on a child that had been diagnosed with ankyloglossia. What is ankyloglossia and how would treatment be documented?

Ankyloglossia, more commonly referred to as "tongue tied," is a condition in which the lingual frenum is short and attached to the tip of the tongue, making normal speech difficult.

The available procedure code is:

D7960 frenulectomy – also known as frenectomy or frenotomy – separate procedure not incidental to another procedure
Removal or release of mucosal and muscle elements of buccal, labial or lingual frenum that is associated with a pathological condition, or interferes with proper oral development or treatment.

18. **A patient presents with a small sialolith in his right Wartons duct. Utilizing non-surgical manipulation which included dilatation and manual manipulation the stone was removed. How would you code for the removal of the stone?**

The correct procedure code is:

D7979 non-surgical sialolithotomy

19. **A restorative dentist refers a patient to your office for evaluation and removal of a broken retaining screw in an implant that you placed two years prior. You are able to remove the screw without damaging the implant. What would the proper code for this procedure be?**

Use the following code to correctly document this procedure:

D6096 remove broken implant retaining screw

20. **An orthodontist refers a patient to the oral surgeon because he would like to accelerate orthodontic movement, and by modifying the alveolus enable teeth to move into areas with limited bone. You determine that a corticotomy would be the appropriate treatment to enable the desired orthodontic movement. How would you code for this procedure?**

The proper code(s) for this procedure depends on the number and location of teeth involved and would be either:

D7296 corticotomy – one to three teeth or tooth spaces, per quadrant

or **D7297 corticotomy – one to three teeth or tooth spaces, per quadrant**

Note: When the involved teeth cross the mid-line two quadrant codes must be reported.

Summary

Oral and maxillofacial surgery cases use codes from many different categories of service, as well as from the CPT medical codes, and requires a step-by-step approach to coding. With time, practice and patience, it will get easier to code for what you do.

Contributor Biography

James E. Mercer, D.D.S. is a board certified oral and maxillofacial surgeon practicing in Columbia, SC since 1988. He is a graduate of Vanderbilt University and The Ohio State University College of Dentistry. He completed a one-year general practice residency, a 2-year research fellowship and his 4-year specialty training in Oral and Maxillofacial Surgery at the Medical College of Georgia at Augusta University.

Dr. Mercer is a past chairman of the ADA's Council on Dental Benefit Programs and has been active in code maintenance nationally since 2003. He continues to be active in the tripartite and is currently a member of the American Association of Oral and Maxillofacial Surgeon's Committee on Health Care Policy, Coding, and Reimbursement representing them on the Code Maintenance Committee, the Dental Quality Alliance, and the SNODENT Maintenance Committee.

Chapter 11.
D8000 – D8999 Orthodontics

By Stephen Robirds, D.D.S.

Introduction

The total number of codes in the Orthodontics category of service is fewer than most other categories. For example, in CDT 2019 there are 22 codes in Orthodontics and 83 in Restorative. The reason for this concise set of codes is that some aspects of an orthodontics case involve procedures (e.g., radiographs) that are documented and reported using CDT codes found in other categories of service.

The purpose of an orthodontic procedure is to reposition teeth in a dental arch and influence skeletal and muscular changes in the oral and maxillofacial complex. This restores health, occlusion, esthetics, or any combination to an acceptable treatment result. Acceptability is to be determined by both the patient (or the patient's parent or guardian) and the treating doctor.

To code for any of these procedures, dentists and their teams must know what they are trying to accomplish in the first place. What is the end result you desire? Are you just expanding a maxillary arch form or is this part of a broader plan to correct the bite and align the teeth? Is it your ultimate goal to simply close a diastema or close space to create an occlusion prior to orthognathic surgery?

In Orthodontics, it is prudent to begin with the end in mind.

Key Definitions and Concepts

Primary Dentition: The stage during which the deciduous (or "baby") teeth erupt and are present. Typically, orthodontic treatment does not begin prior to complete eruption of the deciduous dentition and the permanent first molars are usually in the process of erupting or have fully erupted. The age of a patient can vary based on development, but usually ranges from ages five to eight.

Transitional Dentition: The stage where the patient still has some deciduous teeth remaining and permanent teeth are emerging. The deciduous cuspids and molars are losing root structure and should be exfoliating during this stage. Age, again, can vary, but typically ranges from nine to twelve years old.

Adolescent Dentition: The stage where deciduous teeth are gone and permanent teeth are erupting or have fully erupted with the exception of the third molars. The patient is still in a growing phase, possibly pre-pubertal or in the process of puberty. Body changes at this time can be dramatic, including extensive growth of the oral-maxillofacial complex. Adolescent dentition typically occurs during ages twelve to fifteen, depending upon the sex of the patient as males and females do mature at different rates.

Adult Dentition: This final stage is the full permanent dentition with little or no patient growth remaining. Third molars, if present, are usually erupted unless there is lack of space for eruption or the teeth are malposed.

Limited Orthodontic Treatment: The category of orthodontic treatment that involves a specific, defined, and limited scope of treatment. An example would be a tooth in crossbite or one that needs guidance during eruption. Limited treatment may not necessarily involve the entire dentition and can be done at any of the stages of dental development.

Codes exist for each stage of development:

- D8010 for the primary dentition
- D8020 for the transitional dentition
- D8030 for the adolescent dentition
- D8040 for the permanent dentition

Limited orthodontic treatment could involve palatal expansion or be as simple singular tooth movement with a retainer. Typically, limited coding can be used to report treatment using simple appliances and simple movements that are directed at improving a specific problem for the patient.

Interceptive Orthodontic Treatment: Treatment performed under this category should only be coded for treatment done during the primary dentition (D8050) or transitional dentition (D8060) stages of dental development.

The three main considerations for this type of treatment are as follows:

- Is there enough room for full eruption of the permanent dentition?
- Are there any concerns about the patient's bite (malocclusion)?
- Can these concerns be improved or corrected with early intervention?

Diagnostic records are important, but the extent to which they are necessary to accurately diagnose the case can vary. Treatment modalities are likely to vary depending on the situation and severity, but often are appliances that don't involve braces. A localized area on one of the arches, one entire arch or both arches may be involved. The idea behind interceptive treatment is to greatly improve issues in these earlier stages of development that simplify or possibly eliminate the need for comprehensive treatment later on. Typical examples may include palatal expansion, appliances to gain or maintain space, or appliances designed to moderate or guide skeletal growth of an individual. In these examples treatment may involve headgear, a Herbst appliance or other growth modifiers.

Comprehensive Orthodontic Treatment: This is the most involved treatment care an orthodontist can provide. It includes careful diagnosis and treatment planning including detailed orthodontic records. It involves correction of the patient's dentofacial issues including any skeletal, muscular, and/or dental disharmony issues. Comprehensive treatment can be provided during the transitional (D8070), adolescent (D8080), or permanent (D8090) dentition stage of dental development. Treatment may include a multi-disciplinary approach and involve treatment or consultation with other dental providers such as oral surgeons and periodontists.

Treatment may also include medical specialty providers such as speech therapists, ENT physicians, etc. This is not to be confused with medically necessary orthodontic cases which are in a completely separate category. MNOC (Medically Necessary Orthodontic Care) cases, according to the Affordable Care Act, are reported using medical diagnostic coding based on the severity of the case, the age of the patient (under 19 years of age), and medical involvement to correct the patient's overriding health issues.

Changes to This Category

A new code for removal of fixed orthodontic appliances during the course of treatment has been added in CDT 2019:

D8695 removal of fixed orthodontic appliance for reasons other than completion of treatment

This code will be used to report removal of appliances for a variety of circumstances other than the end of active treatment. Patients may request removal of the appliances in order to undergo a procedure such as an MRI, or may request removal for esthetic reasons such as participation in a wedding, etc. Removal of appliances and placement of retainers at the conclusion of active treatment should be reported using **D8680 orthodontic retention (removal of appliances, construction and placement of retainer(s))**.

Diagnosis Codes – ICD-10-CM

The CDT to ICD tables in Appendix 1 provide appropriate guidance on linkages between often used Orthodontics procedure codes, and diagnosis codes. There are additional ICD-10-CM codes that may be applicable in some situations, or for procedures not listed. These additional codes are in the following table by terms, conditions or anatomy.

Term/Condition/ Anatomy	Code	Definition
Orthodontic exam and evaluation	Z01.89	Encounter for other specified special examinations
Pain	G24.3	Spasmodic torticollis
	G24.4	Idiopathic Orofacial dystonia (Orofacial dyskinesia)
	G44.1	Vascular headache, not elsewhere classified
	G44.201	Tension-type headache, unspecified, intractable
	G44.209	Tension-type headache, unspecified, not intractable
	G44.211	Episodic tension-type headache, intractable
	G44.219	Episodic tension-type headache, not intractable
	G44.221	Chronic tension-type headache, intractable
	G44.229	Chronic tension-type headache, not intractable
	G50.0	Trigeminal neuralgia
	G50.1	Atypical face pain
	H57.10	Ocular pain, unspecified eye
	H57.11	Ocular pain, right eye
	H57.12	Ocular pain, left eye
	H57.13	Ocular pain, bilateral
	M26.62	Arthralgia of the temporomandibular joint
	M54.2	Cervicalgia
	M79.1	Myalgia
	M79.2	Neuralgia and neuritis, unspecified

Term/Condition/ Anatomy	Code	Definition
Migraine – Always check with patient's primary care provider for which migraine code applies.	G43.001	Migraine without aura, not intractable, with status migrainosus
	G43.009	Migraine without aura, not intractable, without status migrainosus
	G43.011	Migraine without aura, intractable, with status migrainosus
	G43.019	Migraine without aura, intractable, without status migrainosus
	G43.101	Migraine with aura, not intractable, with status migrainosus
	G43.109	Migraine with aura, not intractable, without status migrainosus
	G43.111	Migraine with aura, not intractable, with status migrainosus
	G43.119	Migraine with aura, intractable, without status migrainosus
	G43.701	Chronic migraine without aura, not intractable, with status migrainosus
	G43.719	Chronic migraine without aura, not intractable, without status migrainosus
	G43.801	Other migraine, not intractable, with status migrainosus
	G43.809	Other migraine, not intractable, without status migrainosus
	G43.811	Other migraine, intractable, with status migrainosus
	G43.819	Other migraine, intractable, without status migrainosus
	G44.1	Vascular headache, not elsewhere classified
Sleep Apnea	G47.30	Sleep Apnea, unspecified
	G47.31	Primary central sleep apnea
	G47.33	Obstructive sleep apnea
	G47.34	Idiopathic sleep related nonobstructive alveolar hypoventilation
	G47.35	Congenital central alveolar hypoventilation Syndrome
	G47.39	Other sleep apnea
	G47.63	Sleep related bruxism
	G47.8	Other sleep disorders
	G47.9	Sleep disorder, unspecified

Term/Condition/ Anatomy	Code	Definition
Nerve Disorders	G50.8	Other disorders of trigeminal nerve
	G50.9	Disorder of trigeminal nerve, unspecified
	G51.8	Other disorders of facial nerve
	G51.9	Disorder of facial nerve, unspecified
	G52.1	Disorders of glossopharyngeal nerve
Disorders of the Ears	H92.01	Otalgia, right ear
	H92.02	Otalgia, left ear
	H92.03	Otalgia, bilateral
	H92.09	Otalgia, unspecified ear
	H93.11	Tinnitus, right ear
	H93.12	Tinnitus, left ear
	H93.13	Tinnitus, bilateral
	H93.19	Tinnitus, unspecified ear
Larynx	J38.5	Laryngeal spasm
Anomalies of jaw-cranial base relationship	M26.10	Unspecified anomaly of jaw-cranial base relationship
	M26.11	Maxillary asymmetry
	M26.12	Other jaw asymmetry
	M26.19	Other specified anomalies of jaw-cranial base relationship
Anomalies of dental arch relationship	M26.20	Unspecified anomaly of dental arch relationship
	M26.211	Malocclusion, Angle's class I
	M26.212	Malocclusion, Angle's class II
	M26.213	Malocclusion, Angle's class III
	M26.219	Malocclusion, Angle's class, unspecified
	M26.220	Open anterior occlusal relationship (anterior openbite)
	M26.221	Open posterior occlusal relationship (posterior openbite)
	M26.23	Excessive horizontal overlap (overjet)
	M26.24	Reverse articulation, crossbite (anterior or posterior)
	M26.25	Anomalies of interarch distance
	M26.29	Other anomalies of dental arch relationship (midline deviation of dental arch; overbite excessive, deep, horizontal or vertical; posterior lingual occlusion of mandibular teeth)

Term/Condition/ Anatomy	Code	Definition
Anomalies of tooth position	M26.30	Unspecified anomaly of tooth position of fully erupted tooth or teeth
	M26.31	Crowding of fully erupted teeth
	M26.32	Excessive spacing of fully erupted teeth (diastema)
	M26.33	Horizontal displacement of fully erupted tooth or teeth
	M26.34	Vertical displacement of fully erupted tooth or teeth
	M26.35	Rotation of fully erupted tooth or teeth
	M26.36	Insufficient interocclusal distance of fully erupted teeth (ridge)
	M26.37	Excessive interocclusal distance of fully erupted teeth
	M26.39	Other anomalies of tooth position of fully erupted tooth or teeth
Other congenital malformations of skull and face bones	Q18.9	Congenital malformation of face and neck, unspecified
	Q35.1	Cleft hard palate
	Q35.3	Cleft soft palate
	Q35.5	Cleft hard palate with cleft soft palate
	Q35.9	Cleft palate, unspecified
	Q37.0	Cleft hard palate with bilateral cleft lip
	Q37.1	Cleft hard palate with unilateral cleft lip
	Q37.2	Cleft soft palate with bilateral cleft lip
	Q37.3	Cleft soft palate with unilateral cleft lip
	Q37.4	Cleft hard and soft palate with bilateral cleft lip
	Q37.5	Cleft hard and soft palate with unilateral cleft lip
	Q37.8	Unspecified cleft palate with bilateral cleft lip
	Q37.9	Unspecified cleft palate with unilateral cleft lip
	Q38.5	Congenital malformations of palate, not elsewhere classified
	Q38.6	Other congenital malformations of mouth
	Q67.0	Congenital facial asymmetry
	Q67.4	Other congenital deformities of skull, face, and jaw
	Q74.0	Cleidocranial dysostosis/Oculoauricular Dysplasia/OAV
	Q75.0	Craniosynostosis, Pierre Robin Sequence
	Q75.1	Craniofacial dysostosis (Crouzon's Syndrome)
	Q75.2	Hypertelorism

Term/Condition/ Anatomy	Code	Definition
Other congenital malformations of skull and face bones	Q75.3	Macrocephaly
	Q75.4	Mandibulofacial dysostosis Treacher Collins Syndrome
	Q75.5	Oculomandibular dysostosis
	Q75.8	Other specified congenital malformations of skull and face bones
	Q75.9	Congenital malformation of skull and face bones, unspecified
Other specified congenital malformation syndromes affecting multiple systems	Q87.0	Congenital malformation syndromes predominately affecting multiple systems Apert's Syndrome (Acrocephalosyndactyly) Pfeiffer Syndrome (Acrocephalosyndactyly)
	Q87.1	Noonan Syndrome
Turner's Syndrome	Q96.0	Karyotype 45.X
	Q96.1	Karyotype 46.X iso (Xq)
	Q96.2	Karyotype 46, X with abnormal sex chromosome, except iso (Xq)
	Q96.3	Mosaicism, 45,X/46, XX or XY
	Q96.4	Mosaicism, 45, X/other cell line(s) with abnormal sex chromosomes
	Q96.8	Other variants of Turner's Syndrome
	Q96.9	Turner's Syndrome, unspecified
Dislocation of jaw	S03.0XXA	Dislocation of jaw, initial encounter
	S03.0XXD	Dislocation of jaw, subsequent encounter
	S03.0XXS	Dislocation of jaw, sequel
Strains and sprains	S03.4XXA	Sprain of jaw, initial encounter
	S03.4XXD	Sprain of jaw, subsequent encounter
	S03.4XXS	Sprain of jaw, sequela
Miscellaneous	E22.0	Acromegaly and pituitary gigantism
	E23.0	Hypopituitarism (growth hormone deficiency)
	G25.3	Myoclonus
	K14.6	Glossodynia
	M32.10	Systemic lupus erythematosus, organ or system involvement unspecified
	M45.9	Ankylosing spondylitis of unspecified sites in spine

Term/Condition/ Anatomy	Code	Definition
Miscellaneous	M43.6	Torticollis
	R42	Dizziness, (light-headedness)
Diseases of Oral Cavity and Sinuses	K00.0	Anodontia (missing teeth) (Oligodontia)
	K00.1	Hyperdontia (supernumerary teeth)
	K00.2	Abnormalities of size and form
	K00.3	Mottled teeth
	K00.4	Disturbances of tooth formation
	K00.5	Hereditary disturbances in tooth structure, not elsewhere classified
	K00.6	Disturbance of tooth eruption
	K00.8	Other specified disorder of tooth development and eruption
	K00.9	Unspecified disorder of tooth development and eruption
	K01.1	Impacted teeth
	K02.51	Dental caries on pit and fissure surface limited to enamel
	K02.52	Dental caries on pit and fissure surface penetrating into dentin
	K02.53	Dental caries on pit and fissure surface penetrating into pulp
	K02.61	Dental caries on smooth surface limited to enamel
	K02.62	Dental caries on smooth surface penetrating into dentin
	K02.63	Dental caries on smooth surface penetrating into pulp
	K02.7	Dental root caries
	K02.9	Dental caries, unspecified
	K03.5	Ankylosis of teeth
	K03.4	Hypercementosis
	K03.5	Ankylosis of teeth
	K03.9	Other specified diseases of hard tissues of teeth
	K05.00	Acute gingivitis, plaque induced
	K05.01	Acute gingivitis, non-plaque induced
	K05.10	Chronic gingivitis, plaque induced
	K05.11	Chronic gingivitis, non-plaque induced

Term/Condition/ Anatomy	Code	Definition
Diseases of Oral Cavity and Sinuses	K05.20	Aggressive gingivitis, plaque induced
	K05.21	Aggressive gingivitis, non-plaque induced
	K05.22	Aggressive gingivitis, generalized
	K05.30	Chronic periodontitis, unspecified
	K05.31	Chronic periodontitis, localized
	K05.32	Chronic periodontitis, generalized
	K05.4	Periodontitis, juvenile periodontitis
	K05.5	Other periodontal diseases
	K05.6	Periodontal diseases, unspecified
	K06.0	Gingival recession
	K06.1	Gingival enlargement
	K06.9	Disorder of gingiva and edentulous alveolar ridge, unspecified
Loss of Teeth	K08.0	Exfoliation of teeth due to systemic causes
	K08.401	Partial loss of teeth, unspecified cause, class I
	K08.402	Partial loss of teeth, unspecified cause, class II
	K08.403	Partial loss of teeth, unspecified cause, class III
	K08.404	Partial loss of teeth, unspecified cause, class IV
	K08.409	Partial loss of teeth, unspecified cause, unspecified class
	K08.411	Partial loss of teeth, due to trauma, class I
	K08.412	Partial loss of teeth, due to trauma, class II
	K08.413	Partial loss of teeth, due to trauma, class III
	K08.414	Partial loss of teeth, due to trauma, class IV
	K08.419	Partial loss of teeth, due to trauma, unspecified class
	K08.211	Partial loss of teeth, due to periodontal disease, class I
	K08.422	Partial loss of teeth, due to periodontal disease, class II
	K08.423	Partial loss of teeth, due to periodontal disease, class III
	K08.424	Partial loss of teeth, due to periodontal disease, Class IV
	K08.429	Partial loss of teeth, due to periodontal disease, Unspecified class
	K08.431	Partial loss of teeth, due to caries, class I

Term/Condition/ Anatomy	Code	Definition
Loss of Teeth	K08.432	Partial loss of teeth, due to caries, class II
	K08.433	Partial loss of teeth, due to caries, class III
	K08.434	Partial loss of teeth, due to caries, class IV
	K08.439	Partial loss of teeth, due to caries, unspecified class
Major anomalies of jaw size	M26.00	Unspecified anomaly of jaw size
	M26.01	Maxillary hyperplasia
	M26.02	Maxillary hypoplasia
	M26.03	Mandibular hyperplasia
	M26.04	Mandibular hypoplasia
	M26.05	Macrogenia
	M26.06	Microgenia
	M26.07	Excessive tuberosity of jaw (entire maxillary tuberosity)
	M26.09	Other specified anomalies of jaw size
Dentofacial functional abnormalities	M26.50	Dentofacial functional abnormalities, unspecified
	M26.51	Abnormal jaw closure
	M26.52	Limited mandibular range of motion
	M26.53	Deviation in opening and closing mandible
	M26.54	Insufficient anterior guidance
	M26.55	Centric occlusion maximum intercuspation discrepancy
	M26.56	Non-working side interference
	M26.57	Lack of posterior occlusal support
	M26.59	Other dentofacial functional abnormalities
Temporomandibular joint disorders	M26.60	Temporomandibular joint disorder, unspecified
	M26.61	Adhesions and ankylosis of temporomandibular joint
	M26.62	Arthralgia of temporomandibular joint
	M26.63	Articular disc disorder of temporomandibular joint
	M26.69	Other specified disorders of temporomandibular joint
Dental alveolar anomalies	M26.70	Unspecified alveolar anomaly
	M26.71	Alveolar maxillary hyperplasia
	M26.72	Alveolar mandibular hyperplasia
	M26.73	Alveolar maxillary hypoplasia

Term/Condition/ Anatomy	Code	Definition
Dental alveolar anomalies	M26.74	Alveolar mandibular hypoplasia
	M26.79	Other specified alveolar anomalies
	M26.81	Anterior soft tissue impingement
	M26.82	Posterior soft tissue impingement
	M26.89	Other dentofacial anomalies
	M26.9	Dentofacial anomaly, unspecified
Other diseases/ disorders of jaws	M27.0	Developmental disorders of jaws
	M27.2	Inflammatory conditions of jaws
	M27.8	Other specified diseases of jaws
	M27.9	Diseases of jaw, unspecified
Down's Syndrome	Q90 codes	Contact patient's primary care provider to determine the correct code
Arthritis and other diseases	M06.9	Rheumatoid arthritis, unspecified
	M08.00	Juvenile rheumatoid arthritis of unspecified site
	A69.20	Lyme disease, unspecified
	L40.52	Psoriatric arthritis mutilans
	L40.54	Psoriatic juvenile arthropathy
	L40.59	Other psoriatic arthropathy
Disorders of Synovium, Tendon, Bursa	M65.9	Synovitis and tenosynovitis, unspecified
Disorders of Muscle, Ligament, Fascia, Soft Tissue	M24.20	Disorder of ligament, unspecified site
	M35.7	Hypermobility syndrome
	M60.9	Myositis, unspecified
	M62.40	Contracture of muscle, unspecified site
	M62.81	Muscle weakness (generalized)
	M62.838	Other muscle spasm
	M79.1	Myalgia

Term/Condition/ Anatomy	Code	Definition
Fractures Last character legend: A = initial encounter D = subsequent encounter S = sequela G = subsequent encounter for fracture with delayed healing K = subsequent encounter with nonunion A fracture not indicated in the patient record as open or closed should be coded to closed.	S02.2XXA	Fracture of nasal bones, initial encounter for closed fracture
	S02.2XXB	Fracture of nasal bones, initial encounter for open fracture
	S02.400A	Malar fracture unspecified, initial encounter for closed fracture
	S02.400B	Malar fracture, unspecified, initial encounter for open fracture
	S02.401A	Maxillary fracture, unspecified, initial encounter for closed fracture
	S02.401B	Maxillary fracture, unspecified, initial encounter for open fracture
	S02.402A	Fracture of zygoma bones, unspecified, initial encounter for closed fracture
	S02.402B	Fracture of zygoma bones, unspecified, initial encounter for open fracture
	S02.411A	LaForte I fracture, initial encounter for closed fracture
	S02.411B	LaForte I fracture, initial encounter for open fracture
	S02.412A	LaForte II fracture, initial encounter for closed fracture
	S02.412B	LaForte II fracture, initial encounter for open fracture
	S02.413A	LaForte III fracture, initial encounter for closed fracture
	S02.413B	LaForte III fracture, initial encounter for open fracture
	S02.42XA	Fracture of alveolus of maxilla, initial encounter for closed fracture
	S02.42XB	Fracture of alveolus of maxilla, initial encounter for open fracture
	S02.600A	Fracture of unspecified part of body of mandible, initial encounter, closed
	S02.600B	Fracture of unspecified part of body of mandible, initial encounter, open
	S02.609A	Fracture of mandible, unspecified, initial encounter, closed
	S02.609B	Fracture of mandible, unspecified, initial encounter, open
	S02.61XA	Fracture of condylar process of mandible, initial encounter for closed fracture
	S02.61XB	Fracture of condylar process of mandible, initial encounter for open fracture

Term/Condition/ Anatomy	Code	Definition
Fractures Last character legend: A = initial encounter D = subsequent encounter S = sequela G = subsequent encounter for fracture with delayed healing K = subsequent encounter with nonunion A fracture not indicated in the patient record as open or closed should be coded to closed.	S02.62XA	Fracture of subcondylar process of mandible, initial encounter for closed fracture
	S02.62XB	Fracture of subcondylar process of mandible, initial encounter for open fracture
	S02.63XA	Fracture of coronoid process of mandible, initial encounter for closed fracture
	S02.63XB	Fracture of coronoid process of mandible, initial encounter for open fracture
	S02.64XA	Fracture of ramus of mandible, initial encounter for closed fracture
	S02.64XB	Fracture of ramus of mandible, initial encounter for open fracture
	S02.65XA	Fracture of angle of mandible, initial encounter for closed fracture
	S02.65XB	Fracture of angle of mandible, initial encounter for open fracture
	S02.66XA	Fracture of symphysis of mandible, initial encounter for closed fracture
	S02.66XB	Fracture of symphysis of mandible, initial encounter for open fracture
	S02.67XA	Fracture of alveolus of mandible, initial encounter for closed fracture
	S02.67XB	Fracture of alveolus of mandible, initial encounter for open fracture
	S02.69XB	Fracture of mandible of other specified site, initial encounter for open fracture
	S02.8XXA	Fracture of other specified skull bones, initial encounter for closed fracture
	S02.8XXB	Fracture of other specified skull bones, initial encounter for open fracture
	S02.91XA	Fracture of unspecified skull and facial bones, initial encounter, closed
	S02.91XB	Fracture of unspecified skull and facial bones, initial encounter, open
	S02.92XA	Unspecified fracture of facial bones, initial encounter, closed
	S02.92XB	Unspecified fracture of facial bones, initial encounter, open

CODING SCENARIO #1

Class II Malocclusion and Severe Crowding

A 12-year-old patient presents with a Class II malocclusion and severe crowding. The patient just lost her last deciduous tooth. Parents want the teeth straightened and bite corrected. The case has been diagnosed and treatment planned for full upper and lower braces and extraction of all four first bicuspids.

How would you code this treatment?

This case would be coded as **D8080 comprehensive orthodontic treatment of the adolescent dentition** because the patient is still experiencing erupting teeth and growth.

CODING SCENARIO #2

Class I Crowding and Clear Aligners

A 35-year-old patient presents with a Class I crowding situation. The patient does not want fixed appliances (i.e., braces), but will agree to wearing a series of clear, plastic trays to straighten the teeth and improve the esthetics of the case.

How would you code this treatment?

Even though this treatment involves a specific appliance, the case should still be coded as **D8090 comprehensive treatment of the adult dentition**.

CODING SCENARIO #3

Crossbite with Lower Anterior Teeth

A nine-year-old patient's tooth, #8, has erupted into crossbite with the lower anterior teeth. The parents are simply interested in getting the central incisor out of crossbite. Different treatment options were offered to the parents for correction of the problem. After the decision was made, treatment on the central incisor was initiated.

How would you code this treatment?

Since this is treating one particular issue or problem with no serious thought to further treatment later on in the patient's development, this case is best reported using **D8020 limited orthodontic treatment of the transitional dentition**.

CODING SCENARIO #4

Thumb Sucking and Appliances

An eight-year-old patient has a thumb sucking habit that the parents are anxious to stop. An appliance was recommended and placed to aid in halting the habit.

How would you code this procedure?

Coding for appliances to stop harmful habits depends upon the design. For removable appliances the code is **D8210 removable appliance therapy**; for a fixed appliance, **D8220 fixed appliance therapy**.

CODING SCENARIO #5

Removable Retainers to Stabilize Teeth

A patient has completed active treatment and is wearing removable retainers to stabilize the teeth. The retainers are becoming loose and require an appointment for the orthodontist to make adjustments to the appliances.

How would you code this visit?

This visit would be coded using **D8681 removable orthodontic retainer adjustment**.

CODING SCENARIO #6

Claim for Diagnostic Services

A dentist wishes to submit a claim for diagnostic procedures needed to prepare the orthodontic treatment plan for reimbursement by a patient's dental benefits plan.

How would you code this claim?

The claim you submit would list each diagnostic procedure performed, which usually includes:

- A patient examination
- Panoramic, cephalometric and photographic images
- Diagnostic study models

The case would then be submitted by selecting the codes for each of the procedures your office renders, none of which are from the CDT Code's Orthodontics category. Applicable codes in this scenario are from Diagnostics:

D0150 comprehensive oral evaluation – new or established patient

D0330 panoramic radiographic image

D0340 2D radiographic (cephalometric) image – acquisition, measurement and analysis

D0350 oral/facial photographic images obtained intra-orally or extra orally

D0470 diagnostic casts

If your office provides a consultation, don't forget to submit for that component as well by using D9450 case presentation, detailed and extensive treatment planning. Many offices overlook this very important part of reporting treatment planning.

CODING SCENARIO #7

Monitoring Growth and Development

After the initial orthodontic evaluation, many times orthodontists will not feel that orthodontic treatment should begin at that time. They will set an appointment for the patient to return in a few months in order to monitor their growth and development. They will then determine if treatment should begin at that point.

What code should be used to report these future visits?

D8660 pre-orthodontic treatment examination to monitor growth and development

CODING SCENARIO #8

Discontinued Treatment and Removal of Braces

A 10-year-old patient's parents have decided that they would like to discontinue orthodontic treatment. As such, they also wish to have their child's braces removed.

How would you code for this scenario?

D8695 removal of fixed orthodontic appliances for reasons other than completion of treatment

Although it may not be needed, please consider requesting the parents sign a waiver of release for premature removal of braces.

The practice should make a decision about whether to provide retention based on the treatment progress made, and in conjunction with the patient's or parent's treatment wishes. In addition, the practice should ensure that the patient's results to-date are held should the decision be reversed and treatment continues.

CODING SCENARIO #9

Orthodontic Work Up Claim Rejection

A claim for an initial orthodontic workup included diagnostic imaging codes D0272 (two bitewings) and D0340 (2-D cephalometric radiographic image), which were rejected. The third-party payer rejected these submissions, saying that an orthodontic work-up must be reported with code D8665.

The dentist told the payer that D8665 is not a valid CDT code and that HIPAA requires the use of codes published in the CDT manual on a claim submission.

The carrier was adamant that the claim be submitted with the D8665 code, not with D0272 and D0340.

What can be done to correct the third-party payer's position?

The CDT Code is the HIPAA standard for reporting dental procedures, and a claim must include codes from the version in effect on the date of service. D8665 is not now and never has been included in any CDT Code version. The third-party payer may use this code internally for adjudication purposes only. Requiring a dentist to report it instead of the valid codes is a HIPAA violation that should be reported, and the third-party payer faces monetary penalties imposed by the federal government.

HIPAA enforcement falls to the Centers for Medicare and Medicaid Services (CMS), which is where a complaint about this third-party payer should be filed. Complaints may be submitted electronically or on paper. Specific guidance on both processes is available online at:

www.cms.gov/Regulations-and-Guidance/Administrative-Simplification/Enforcements/FileaComplaint.html

Notifying the third-party payer of your intent to file a complaint may be sufficient for it to correct its position. Please contact the ADA for further assistance at 800-621-8099 or *dentalcode@ada.org*.

CODING SCENARIO #10

Removal of Orthodontic Braces and Appliances by General Dentist in an Emergency Situation

A patient with braces has been struck in the face. Since it's an emergency, the patient is rushed to his general dentist. In order to assess and repair the damage, the dentist must remove the patient's braces and appliances.

How would you code for the removal of the patient's braces and appliances?

D8695 removal of fixed orthodontic appliances for reasons other than the completion of treatment

Coding Q&A

1. **Many offices now produce digital versus plaster study models for their cases. What code should be used to report digital study models?**

   Code D0470 should still be used to report fabrication of orthodontic study models. CDT coding is intended to be procedure specific, not modality or technique specific.

2. **Can D0470 diagnostic casts can be used to bill iTero scans used in lieu of diagnostic models?**

   D0470 diagnostic casts may still be used when digital scans are used in lieu of fabrication of plaster models. Dental codes are procedure specific and not technique/modality specific.

3. **What code or codes should be used to report multiple stages of orthodontic treatment?**

   It is best to use limited coding for the initial phase of orthodontic treatment when you are treating only a portion of the dentition (e.g., treatment of crossbite with an expansion appliance). Interceptive treatment is often the coding for initial orthodontic care that typically is followed later in the patient's development with comprehensive (full) treatment.

4. **What are the differences between limited, interceptive, and comprehensive codes and how should they be used?**

   Limited (D8010-D8040) and Interceptive (D8050-D8060) codes are generally used to report less complex cases or initial stages of treatment. Comprehensive (D8070-D8090) codes are generally reserved for more complex cases.

5. **What code should be used to report treatment using clear aligners?**

   In most cases, when clear aligner therapy is used, the entire dentition is being treated. It is best to use comprehensive coding, modified by the appropriate stage of dental development to submit this case.

6. **When should an orthodontic practice use D8999 unspecified orthodontic procedure, by report?**

   This code should be used sparingly and only when there is absolutely no other coding strategy available. In most cases another code can be found that will adequately and appropriately report the procedure performed. If the code is used, make certain that the claim is accompanied by a narrative report to describe the patient's condition, the need for treatment and the treatment provided.

7. **Often times when orthodontic cases are completed, the orthodontist may wish to put final touches on the case to perfect the end result by slightly altering the shape of a tooth or teeth. What code should be used?**

   The code most often used to report slight revisions to tooth shape is **D9971 odontoplasty, 1-2 teeth; includes removal of enamel projections**.

8. **What code should be used to report space maintainers: space maintenance codes or interceptive coding? How should holding arches be reported?**

   The appropriate space maintenance code (D1510; D1516-D1517; D1520; D1526-D1527; or D1575) should be used if only a single space is being held. Treatment with holding arches is best reported using limited treatment procedure codes (D8010-D8040) if several spaces are being held.

9. **A patient has been placed on recall appointments every four months to monitor growth and development and to determine the best time to start orthodontic treatment. How should these appointments be recorded?**

   These appointments should be reported using **D8660 pre-orthodontic treatment examination to monitor growth and development**.

10. **A patient is being seen monthly for routine orthodontic treatment. How are these appointments coded?**

    These appointments are coded using **D8670 periodic orthodontic treatment visit**.

11. **A patient has lost her retainer and it must be replaced. What code would you use?**

    Replacement of lost or broken retainers is coded using D8692 replacement of lost or broken retainer.

12. **An orthodontic patient is attending college in a different city than where he lived when he started his treatment. The patient locates an orthodontist in the college town to continue treatment. How should services from an orthodontist other than the originally treating orthodontist be coded?**

    Services from an orthodontist other than the originally treating orthodontist should be coded **D8690 orthodontic treatment (alternative billing to a contract fee)**.

13. **A patient has a palatal expander that has come loose due to a broken expansion arm. The appliance is removed, repaired, and re-cemented. How would you code the repairs?**

    For repairs of orthodontic appliances (excluding brackets and standard fixed appliances), use code **D8691 repair of orthodontic appliance**.

14. **A bonded retainer on the lingual aspect of the lower six anterior teeth has come loose and must be re-bonded. How would you code for re-bonding this retainer?**

    The code for re-cementing or re-bonding fixed retainers is **D8693 re-cement or re-bond fixed retainer**.

15. **A bonded retainer has come loose and the wire is bent out of shape. The retainer must be removed, reshaped properly, and rebonded. What code would you use for repair and reattachment?**

    Use code **D8694 repair of fixed retainers, includes reattachment**.

16. A patient has undergone diagnostic procedures, has had their consultation, and has agreed on their treatment plan. The patient is ready to begin orthodontic treatment. To prepare adequate space for orthodontic bands to be fitted around some teeth, separators are placed. Can placement of separators be considered as the official start of orthodontic treatment?

Placement of separators does not signify the start of orthodontic treatment. The official start of orthodontic treatment begins when appliances are delivered (Herbst, etc.) or placed for the patient (braces, etc.).

17. When should adolescent coding be used versus adult coding?

Adolescent coding should be used when the patient involved is approximately 11 to 13 years of age, presents with adult dentition and is expected to undergo further growth. Adult coding should be considered when the patient has full adult dentition (may or may not have third molars present), is approximately 17 years of age or older and is not expected to experience additional growth.

18. How does a dentist bill for a tongue presser appliance?

D8210 removable appliance therapy

D8220 fixed appliance therapy

19. How do I bill for accelerated orthodontic treatment cases?

Even if the treatment time is less than the traditional standard treatment time, the same coding rules apply. The codes you use also depend on whether the treatment is comprehensive or limited. The age of the patient is a factor, too.

If the full dentition is being engaged, the recommended code is:

D8080 comprehensive orthodontic treatment of the adolescent dentition

or **D8090 comprehensive orthodontic treatment of adult dentition**

If not all dentition is engaged in the treatment, the recommended code is:

D8030 limited orthodontic treatment of the primary dentition

or **D0840 limited orthodontic treatment of the adult dentition**

20. The practice has had numerous requests for the orthodontist's tax identification number when the office does not accept assignment of benefits. The office is concerned that, if the tax identification number is supplied, it will result in incorrect or even perhaps duplicate information being supplied to the Internal Revenue Service via a 1099 form. What can be done?

The purpose in providing the practice tax identification number (TIN) is for the payer to report earned income to the IRS. For dentists who do not accept assignment of benefits there is no valid legal reason for supplying the information as the payer has not paid the dentist for services rendered. The dentist should contact their own legal advisor regarding appropriate next steps, which may include requesting the payer for documentation that establishes the legal basis for the TIN request.

Summary

To properly use orthodontics codes, it is best to understand what you are trying to accomplish as your final result. How complex is the treatment plan? How comprehensive is the treatment plan? You should also consider that many dental insurance plans have limited lifetime coverage for orthodontic treatment. The practitioner must be very careful in determining what codes to use and when to maximize the most effective coverage for the patient.

Contributor Biography

Stephen Robirds, D.D.S. has been a practicing orthodontist in Austin, Texas since 1982. He began work with ADA CDT code revision process in 2006 when he became a member of the Council on Orthodontic Healthcare of the American Association of Orthodontists. He is currently the council's consultant on all matters relating to dental insurance and is a member of the ADA's Code Maintenance Committee.

Chapter 12.
D9000 – D9999
Adjunctive General Services

By Charles D. Stewart, D.M.D.

Introduction

"Adjunctive" refers to any treatment or service delivered with a primary treatment that increases the primary treatment's efficacy, or to assist with completion or reporting of the primary treatment. In other words, adjunctive treatment or therapy is generally a secondary treatment or activity in addition to the primary therapy.

The Adjunctive General Services category is often searched when an appropriate CDT code can't be found in any of the 11 other CDT Code sections. The category is unique, with CDT codes for clinical services, non-clinical services, and for administrative or compliance requirements and services. This uniqueness has led many to describe this section as a catch-all, with both procedures and services that don't quite fit elsewhere. Many of the codes in this section are for care or administrative activities that happen outside of the mouth, but occur in the practice administrative office or location setting.

Key Definitions and Concepts

Anesthesia: A patient's level of consciousness is determined by the patient's response to the drugs or medications administered, not the route of the anesthetic agent administration. State dental boards regulate the use of anesthesia techniques. The ADA House of Delegates adopted and has published an anesthesia policy and guidelines, which are available at *ADA.org/en/member-center/oral-health-topics/anesthesia-and-sedation*. Anesthesia has many CDT definitions and applications such as local, regional, deep sedation, general anesthesia, etc.

Key Definitions and Concepts

Consultation: In a dental setting, a diagnostic service provided by a dentist or other licensed dental professional where the dentist, patient, or other parties (e.g., another dentist, physician, or legal guardian) discuss the patient's dental needs, conditions and proposed treatment modalities.

Medicament: Substance or combination of substances intended to be pharmacologically active, specially prepared to be prescribed, dispensed or administered by authorized personnel to prevent or treat diseases in humans or animals. This can be an agent that promotes recovery from an injury or ailment. Also referred to as a medicine.

Microabrasion: Mechanical and chemical removal of a small amount of tooth structure to eliminate superficial enamel discoloration defects. Utilizes chemical solutions and pumice to remove thin layers of tooth enamel, removing yellow, white and brown spots, stains and discolorations on the teeth.

Palliative: Action that relieves pain without dealing with the cause of the condition.

Parenteral: A technique of administration in which the drug bypasses the gastrointestinal (GI) tract. Examples of parenteral administration may include intramuscular (IM), intravenous (IV), intranasal (IN), submucosal (SM), subcutaneous (SC) or intraosseous (IO).

Teledentisty, Asynchronous: Also known as "store-and-forward," involves transmission of recorded health information to a dentist, who uses the information to evaluate a patient's condition or render a service outside of a real-time or live interaction. Such transmitted information can include radiographs, photographs, video, digital impressions, digital models and photomicrographs of patients. Transmission is through a secure electronic communications system.

Teledentistry, Synchronous: Also referred to as live video or real-time, synchronous teledentistry involves live, two-way interaction between a person (patient, caregiver, or provider) and a dentist using audiovisual telecommunications technology.

Changes to This Category

There are several code changes in this category in CDT 2019.

Adjunctive – Unclassified Treatment

This is the first CDT version that includes a code for a physical therapy procedure, one that pertains to treatment of TMJ symptoms or dysfunction – various modalities that could only be reported with D7899 unspecified TMD therapy, by report. The new code recognizes that TMJ treatment need not be limited to appliance therapy or surgical procedures.

D9130 temporomandibular joint dysfunction – non-invasive physical therapies
Therapy including but not limited to massage, diathermy, ultrasound, or cold application to provide relief from muscle spasms, inflammation or pain, intending to improve freedom of motion and joint function. This should be reported on a per session basis.

This new code is to be reported on a per session basis. The Code Maintenance Committee determined that this CDT code entry should not define a session, or the number of sessions that may be delivered on a specific date of service.

Many dental benefit plans do not cover TMJ treatments but some medical benefit plans do.

Adjunctive – Anesthesia

Following the CDT 2018 changes made in this category, it was determined that the existing CDT code D9219 needed to be modified to be inclusive of moderate sedation. As listed in the definition of anesthesia noted earlier in this chapter, a patient's level of consciousness is determined by the patient's response to the drugs or medications administered, not the route of the anesthetic agent administration. For this reason, code D9219 was broadened to include the evaluation for moderate sedation, in addition to deep sedation or general anesthesia.

D9219 evaluation for moderate sedation, deep sedation or general anesthesia

In the discussion of this proposed revision, the Code Maintenance Committee agreed that the evaluation for these anesthesia services did not differ for any of the above levels of sedation or anesthesia.

Adjunctive – Drugs

Headlines in recent years have been riddled with news of the opioid epidemic. This epidemic has resulted in new laws and regulations. In response to this crisis, the American Dental Association has released an interim opioids policy, which defines the role dentists play in the provision of opioids. This new CDT code, effective January 1, 2019 provides a means to document delivery of non-opioid medications that manage post-surgical pain (e.g., as may be encounter after third molar removal).

D9613 infiltration of sustained release therapeutic drug – single or multiple sites
Infiltration of a sustained release pharmacologic agent for long acting surgical site pain control. Not for local anesthesia purposes.

The use of medicaments such as the above have historically been reported using CDT code D9610. With the new code it will be possible to identify the intent of the medication used, and it would be possible to track the usage of these medications to determine the impact this has on helping control the opioid crisis. With this new code, it is expected that the need for a prescription for an opioid medication following oral surgical procedures can be limited to an emergency prescription only, if any at all.

Adjunctive – Miscellaneous Services – Occlusal Guards

Changes to these procedures had been presented for consideration in past cycles of the code maintenance process. The intent of these changes was in response to concerns that there is not one type of occlusal guard, with every type of guard having varying fees associated with the fabrication of the appliance.

~~**D9940 occlusal guard, by report**~~
~~Removable dental appliances, which are designed to minimize the effects of bruxism (grinding) and other occlusal factors.~~

This deletion is appropriate based on the addition of the followinq three new codes:

D9944 occlusal guard – hard appliance, full arch
Removable dental appliance designed to minimize the effects of bruxism or other occlusal factors. Not to be reported for any type of sleep apnea, snoring or TMD appliances

These appliances are for hard material, full arch. Usually only one appliance is fabricated for the treatment of bruxism or other occlusal factors. Appliances for treatment of sleep apnea or TMJ symptoms should not be reported with this code.

D9945 occlusal guard – soft appliance, full arch
Removable dental appliance designed to minimize the effects of bruxism or other occlusal factors. Not to be reported for any type of sleep apnea, snoring or TMD appliances.

These appliances are for soft material, full arch. Usually only one appliance is fabricated for the treatment of bruxism or other occlusal factors. Appliances for treatment of sleep apnea or TMJ symptoms should not be reported with this code.

D9946 occlusal guard – hard appliance, partial arch
Removable dental appliance designed to minimize the effects of bruxism or other occlusal factors. Provides only partial occlusal coverage such as anterior deprogrammer. Not to be reported for any type of sleep apnea, snoring or TMD appliances.

These appliances are for hard material, partial arch. Usually only one appliance is fabricated for the treatment of bruxism or other occlusal factors. This has been referred to as an anterior deprogrammer or anterior disclusion device. Appliances for treatment of sleep apnea or TMJ symptoms should not be reported with this code.

Adjunctive – Non-Clinical Procedures

This growing subcategory can be called administrative codes or housekeeping codes, many of which address legal processes or requirements and their reporting. Procedures in this category include the reporting of office procedures (tax, missed or cancelled appointments) and the codes added in CDT 2017 for case management and those in CDT 2018 for teledentistry.

The additions in CDT 2019 are:

D9961 duplicate/copy patient's records

This new code is unique as it represents a method of documenting that indeed the patient records have been copied or duplicated. Many states require dental providers to copy or duplicate patient records upon request, and many of those states have defined what can be charged for this service, if anything.

D9990 certified translation or sign-language services per visit

Certified translation or sign-language services are required services under many federal or state laws, programs or benefit plans. This new code allows a practitioner to report the use of a certified interpreter or translator. Federal or state laws may specify what may be charged and will define the scope of what services are to be provided. CMC discussion of this new code, prior to its acceptance, addressed reporting the time period or unit for the service. The committee concluded that reporting on a per visit basis is appropriate.

Diagnosis Codes – ICD-10-CM

The CDT to ICD tables in Appendix 1 provide appropriate guidance on linkages between often used Adjunctive General Services procedure codes, and diagnosis codes.

ICD codes also aid in establishing "medical necessity," which is especially pertinent when claims are submitted to medical benefit plans and Medicare.

Note: The ADA's online Glossary of Dental Clinical and Administrative Terms defines "medically necessary care" as:

> The reasonable and appropriate diagnosis, treatment, and follow-up care (including supplies, appliances and devices) as determined and prescribed by qualified, appropriate health care providers in treating any condition, illness, disease, injury, or birth developmental malformations. Care is medically necessary for the purpose of: controlling or eliminating infection, pain, and disease; and restoring facial configuration or function necessary for speech, swallowing or chewing.

"Medical necessity" is not static. The prudent approach is to anticipate that a claim for dental services will be filed against a patient's medical benefit plan or Medicare, and determine and document the patient's diagnosis at every visit. Even if there is no such claim filed, the patient's dental record will be more robust by inclusion of codified diagnostic information.

Coding Scenarios

CODING SCENARIO #1

Denture Cleaning

The patient presents with a chief complaint of hot and cold sensitivity of teeth #22 and #27. She has a full upper denture and partial lower denture. The initial treatment plan is to clean the dentures and take four periapical radiographic images of all remaining lower teeth. Upon viewing the images, the dentist sees no caries and no periapical pathology for teeth #22 and #27. Both have significant gingival recession with deep erosion at the gingival margin of #22. The dentist performs desensitizing treatment for tooth #27 and a cervical resin restoration for tooth #22.

How do you code this care?

D0140 limited oral evaluation – problem focused

D0220 intraoral periapical first radiographic image

D0230 intraoral periapical each additional periapical image

This procedure is reported three times as this is the number of additional images (four total images exposed).

D9910 application of desensitizing medicament

This procedure is reported for tooth #27.

D9911 application of desensitizing resin for cervical and/or root surface

This procedure is reported for tooth #22.

D9932 cleaning and inspection of complete denture, maxillary

D9935 cleaning and inspection of removable partial denture, mandibular

CODING SCENARIO #2

Anesthesia Complications

A patient, referred by a general dentist, is scheduled for surgical removal of third molars. An evaluation for the use of general anesthesia was conducted, resulting in the decision to proceed with the anesthetic and surgery upon obtaining the appropriate informed consents. After the administration of the anesthetic medication, the patient became combative and the anesthesia and surgery were abandoned.

How would you code this care?

D9219 evaluation for moderate sedation, deep sedation or general anesthesia

D9222 deep sedation/general anesthesia – first 15 minutes

In the above clinical scenario, it would be recommended to include a narrative along with the above codes. Copies of the anesthesia records may also be recommended for verification of the time of anesthesia. Since there was no surgical procedure completed, the narrative would explain the surgery was abandoned due to the patient's combative reaction to the anesthesia.

CODING SCENARIO #3

Incomplete Extraction

An emergency patient in pain requires a molar to be extracted. The dentist prefers to refer this patient to an oral surgeon. No oral surgeons have appointment availability, and to assist the patient and relieve the source of their pain, the general dentist agrees to remove the molar. As no good deed goes unpunished, the molar shatters and the general dentist is unable to remove the entire tooth.

Is there a way to report a partial extraction or incomplete extraction?

There is no CDT code to document a partial or incomplete transaction, which means that the situation would be documented with:

D7999 unspecified oral surgery procedure, by report

Should the patient require additional services, such as temporary pain relief prior to being seen by an oral surgeon, the available code is:

D9110 palliative (emergency) treatment of dental pain – minor procedure

CODING SCENARIO #4

Occlusal Equilibration

The patient says her spouse hears loud grinding sounds at night, but says she has no pain in her jaws or joint area. However, the patient reports that she does have difficulty chewing food, and that the teeth seem to "chatter" when chewing.

Based on this information and oral evaluation, the dentist determined that the patient needed her bite adjusted.

How would you code the "bite adjustment" procedure?

Occlusal equilibration, also known as occlusal adjustment, refers to the reshaping of the occlusal surfaces of teeth to create a harmonious contact relationship between the upper and lower teeth. One of the following codes should be used, with selection based on the procedure's extent:

D9951 occlusal adjustment – limited

or **D9952 occlusal adjustment – complete**

If the occlusal equilibration is associated with or to accommodate the placement of a restoration or prosthesis, the billing of the equilibration may be considered incidental to the restoration or prosthesis.

CODING SCENARIO #5

Dry Socket

A student came home from college to have his third molars removed. He returned to college, with complaints of worsening pain in the mandibular extraction sites. He sought the care of a local dentist in the college town. The dentist examined the patient and diagnosed condensing osteitis, or dry socket, in the mandibular extraction sites.

How would you code this care?

A dry socket is localized inflammation of the tooth socket following extraction due to failure of the development of a blood clot or the loss of the blood clot with resultant osteitis. The condition is very painful and characterized by bad breath and an unpleasant smell and taste in the mouth. The procedure could be coded as either:

D9930 treatment of complications (post-surgical) – unusual circumstances, by report

or **D9110 palliative (emergency) treatment of dental pain – minor procedure**

D0140 limited oral evaluation – problem focused would be appropriate in addition to one of the above CDT codes as the dentist did perform a limited oral evaluation in determining the source of the chief complaint.

CODING SCENARIO #6

Gingival Irritation Around a Partially Erupted Third Molar

A patient reported to the dentist with a complaint of inflammation and pain from the gums around an unerupted third molar. The patient complained that food was getting stuck in the flap of tissue. The dentist evaluated the area and diagnosed pericornitis. The dentist irrigated the area to remove and flush out the trapped food.

How would you code this care?

D0140 limited oral evaluation – problem focused

and **D9110 palliative (emergency) treatment of dental pain – minor procedure**

This is typically reported on a "per visit" basis for emergency treatment of dental pain.

Using D9110 is appropriate as the patient did report to the dental office on an emergency basis with the complaint of pain around the third molar. The minor procedure was the irrigation of the food entrapment. D9110 does not define what procedure needs to be performed to qualify nor that the procedure be completed.

There are some that feel the irrigation could be coded using "D4921 gingival irrigation – per quadrant." This code's descriptor notes that the procedure is for irrigation of gingival pockets, which is not the case in this scenario and therefore the reason why D4291 is not applicable.

While on the subject of the D4921, this code is not intended to be used to report the irrigation of a socket following the extraction.

CODING SCENARIO #7

Assessments at a Title I School – A "Real Time" Teledentistry Encounter

(Scenario assumes that the persons and services involved are performing services in accordance and compliance with all local, state, federal laws, rules, and regulations (e.g., dental practice acts or laws).

A hygienist is scheduled to meet with students of a local Title I school in order to assess their potential need for dental treatment. The school does not have dedicated space or equipment for dental assessments, so the hygienist brings a laptop computer and an intraoral camera, as well as a portable dental chair and unit. There is also portable radiographic equipment. This equipment is used to enable information capture and a real-time connection with the dentists via a HIPAA-compliant secure connection that uses encryption technology.

During the visit the hygienist records patient information that includes a clinical examination, perio evaluation, a visual oral cancer examination, and capture of high-quality intraoral diagnostic images. The dentist through this real-time connection sees ten patients exhibiting evidence of the need for immediate or further care (e.g., restorations, prophylaxis, extraction and fluoride application). Several of the students schedule their care at the affiliated brick and mortar dental practice following consultation with their parents.

What CDT codes would be used to document the services provided on the day of this real-time encounter?

In this scenario, patients present for diagnostic and evaluative procedures. The dentist is at a different physical location with complete and immediate access to patient information being captured and the ability to interact vocally and visually with the patient and the hygienist.

The following procedure codes are reported by the oral health or general health practitioner, as applicable, for each patient who received the services described.

D0191 assessment of a patient

D0220 intraoral periapical first radiographic image

D0230 intraoral periapical each additional periapical image

D0350 2D oral/facial photographic image obtained intra-orally or extra-orally

D0351 3D photographic image

Note: The types of diagnostic image (2D or 3D), as well as the number of separate images captured would be determined by the dentist/hygienist to adequately document the clinical condition.

D01xx (oral evaluation CDT code – determined and reported by the dentist)

D9995 teledentistry – synchronous; real-time encounter

Note: D9995 is reported once for each patient, in the same manner as CDT code "D9410 house/extended care facility call" (once per date of service per patient) to document the type of teledentistry interaction in this setting on the date of service.

CODING SCENARIO #8

Screening Services at an Off-Site Setting – A "Store and Forward" Teledentistry Encounter

(Scenario assumes that the persons and services involved are performing services in accordance and compliance with all local, state, federal laws, rules, and regulations (e.g., dental practice acts or laws).

A dental auxiliary in an off-site setting collects a full set of electronic dental records as allowed in the state where the facility is located. These records include radiographs, photographs, charting of dental conditions, health history, consent, and applicable progress notes. This stored information is forwarded to the dentist via a secure HIPAA-compliant connection that uses encryption technology. At a later time, the dentist completes the oral evaluation, diagnosis, and treatment plan.

What CDT codes would be used to document the services provided at the off-site setting?

In this scenario the patient interacts only with the dental auxiliary. The information collected is conveyed to the dentist for diagnosis, evaluation and treatment planning at a later time, and possibly at a different location. This dentist has no live vocal or visual interaction with the patient or dental auxiliary during information collection.

The following procedure codes can be reported, as applicable, for each individual who received the services described:

D0190 screening of a patient

D0220 intraoral periapical first radiographic image

D0230 intraoral periapical each additional periapical image

D0350 2D oral/facial photographic image obtained intra-orally or extra-orally

D0351 3D photographic image

Note: The types of diagnostic image (2D or 3D), as well as the number of separate images captured would be determined by the clinical condition being documented.

D9996 teledentistry – asynchronous; information stored and forwarded to dentist for subsequent review

Note: D9996 is reported once for each patient to document the type of teledentistry interaction in this setting on the date of service.

1. **Who could document and report a D9995 or D9996 CDT code?**

   A dentist who oversees the teledentistry event, and who, via diagnosis and treatment planning, completes the oral evaluation, may report the appropriate teledentistry procedure code. Applicable state regulations may also determine the oral health or general health practitioner who documents and reports these codes.

2. **What documentation should I maintain in my patient records, and what will be needed on a claim submission when reporting teledentistry codes D9995 and D9996?**

   The patient record should include the CDT code that reflects the type of teledentistry encounter, and there may be additional state documentation requirements to satisfy. Treatment records should be very specific and document the scenario in which the encounter occurs. A claim submission must include all required information as described in the completion instructions for the ADA paper claim form and the HIPAA standard electronic dental claim. Some government programs (e.g., Medicaid) may have additional claim reporting requirements.

3. **May I report "D9110 palliative (emergency) treatment of dental pain - minor procedure" and another procedure on the same day?**

   There is no language in the descriptor of D9110 that precludes the reporting of other procedures on the same date of service. However, benefit plan limitations may exclude or not recognize certain combinations of codes performed on the same day.

4. **How may I report local anesthesia as a separate procedure?**

   D9215 local anesthesia in conjunction with operative or surgical procedures is an available code if you wish to report it separately. Benefit plan limitations may exclude separate reimbursement benefits for local anesthesia.

5. **Our office used code "D9610 therapeutic parenteral drug, single administration" to report injection of sedative agents. As of January 1, 2007, D9610 was revised to prohibit the reporting of sedative agents. How should the injection of sedative agents be reported?**

   There is no specific CDT code for injection of a sedative agent. The following code may be reported as its descriptor states the procedure includes non-IV minimal and moderate sedation:

   D9248 non-intravenous conscious sedation

   An alternative is **D9999 unspecified adjunctive procedure, by report**.

6. **Should a specialist who sees a patient referred by a general dentist for an evaluation of a specific problem report the consultation code (D9310) or a problem focused evaluation code (D0140 or D0160)? Also, does it matter if the specialist initiates treatment for the patient on the same visit?**

   Typically, a consultation (D9310) is reported when one dentist refers a patient to another dentist for an opinion or advice on a particular problem encountered by the patient. According to this CDT code's descriptor, the dentist who is consulted may initiate additional diagnostic or therapeutic services for the patient. These services are reported separately by their own unique CDT codes.

   Both D0140 and D0160 are problem focused evaluations and may be reported if the consulting specialist believes either better describes the service provided. Please note that neither of these evaluation procedures' nomenclatures or descriptors contain language that prohibits the consulting specialist from initiating and reporting additional services.

7. **If a practitioner treats more than one patient in one nursing home on one day, is D9410 house/extended care facility call reported per patient or per facility?**

   The descriptor for code D9410 states that it may be reported in addition to separate reporting of services provided to a patient seen at the facility. D9410 may be reported for each patient receiving service at the facility on a given day. However, benefit plan limitations and exclusions may place limits on reimbursement, such as once per facility visit, not per patient.

8. **A patient was complaining of grinding their teeth. The symptoms are worsening as final examinations approach. The dentist makes something called an anterior deprogrammer to provide relief and get this patient through finals. What CDT code should be used to report this?**

   As there is no indication of TMD code D9944 effective with CDT 2019 is appropriate for reporting the services performed.

   D9944 occlusal guard – hard appliance, partial arch

   This code properly represents the described service performed as it notes the device is a "removable dental appliance designed to minimize the effects of bruxism or other occlusal factors." The guard provides partial occlusal coverage as an anterior deprogrammer.

9. **How do I report external bleaching?**

   You may use one of the following codes as applicable based on the extent of the service provided to the patient:

   D9972 external bleaching – per arch – performed in the office

   or **D9973 external bleaching – per tooth**

10. **Are professional strength at-home teeth whitening and bleaching systems delivered in the office reportable under code "D9972 external bleaching – per arch – performed in the office?"**

    D9972 is applicable to in-office service.

    When material is provided to a patient for application at home the following code is applicable:

    D9975 external bleaching for home application, per arch; includes materials and fabrication of custom trays

11. **Is there a code for relining or repairing an occlusal guard?**

    Report code **D9942 repair and/or reline of occlusal guard**.

12. After placing an occlusal guard, the dentist asks patients return for approximately three to four office visits, as needed, to adjust the guard. What procedure code would be used to report visits to adjust the guard?

D9943 occlusal guard adjustment

13. Is there a CDT code for air abrasion?

There is no procedure code specifically for air abrasion.

If the procedure delivered is consistent with the nomenclature and descriptor of **D9970**, that code may be reported. The code and nomenclature is as follows:

D9970 enamel microabrasion
The removal of discolored surface enamel defects resulting from altered mineralization or decalcification of the superficial enamel layer. Submit per treatment visit.

Summary

The adjunctive general services codes are an important part of a dental care treatment plan because they can increase or influence the first treatment's efficacy. In an ever-changing healthcare environment, dentistry will continue to evolve and develop more ways to measure and increase the efficacy of our treatments.

For example, teledentistry provides the opportunity and means for a patient to receive services when the patient is in one physical location and a dentist overseeing the delivery of those services is in another location. With the addition of the CDT codes for teledentistry, access to care has been influenced and the potential to bring dental care to patients in areas without a dentist is now a reality.

Equally exciting is the opportunity afforded by the addition of a CDT code for the infiltration of sustained release therapeutic drug – single or multiple sites. This code, D9613, is new for CDT 2019 can impact and potentially eliminate the need for an opioid prescription. With education of both patients and dental providers, this newly recognized procedure can influence one of the first exposures to an opioid helping to address the current opioid epidemic.

The Adjunctive General Services codes will be the one category in the CDT that will have future changes to reflect the evolution of issues in the regulatory and compliance environment.

Contributor Biography

Charles D. Stewart, D.M.D. is currently President, CEO and Chairman of the Board of Directors for Aetna Dental of California, Inc. He is also National Director, Dental Networks, for Aetna Inc. He is currently Chairman of California Association of Dental Plans (CADP) Quality Management Committee, member of the CADP Board of Directors, and the lead instructor for CADP's quality assurance consultant certification courses. Dr. Stewart is credited with the development and implementation of the CADP computerized shared quality assurance assessment warehouse program. He lectures nationally on various topics related to the Dental Benefits Industry such as, coding, fraud prevention and quality assurance issues. In addition to the above, Dr. Stewart maintains a private practice on evenings and weekends. He is affiliated with the ADA, CDA and San Fernando Valley Dental Society, and is a member of the American Academy of Oral and Maxillofacial Radiology. Dr Stewart is a graduate of Oral Roberts University School of Dentistry.

Chapter 13. Dental Benefits: What Every Dentist Should Know

By ADA Staff
Center for Dental Benefits, Coding and Quality, Practice Institute

This chapter addresses facets of a dental practice's business side, things a dentist should be aware of that will help anticipate or resolve problems. Topics covered include ascertaining a patient's benefits, becoming a participating dentist, claim processing problems and audits. The chapter concludes with links to additional related resources available from the American Dental Association.

Dental Benefit Coverage

The majority of patients with private dental benefits coverage have their plans provided by employers or unions. Employers offer dental plans to help attract and retain employees and to help employees maintain good oral health. However, most dental plans are not designed to cover all dental procedures and many procedures require the patient to meet a deductible or incur a high co-insurance payment. It is very important for dental offices to explain to their patients that a dental benefit plan is actually not insurance but simply a benefit. Thus, it is essential to educate your patients about costs and recommend they take their dental benefit grievances to their employer's human resources department when necessary.

Making the Decision to Participate with a Managed Care Plan

Making the decision to sign a managed care contract is one of the most important business decisions a dentist may make. When you sign a contract, you make promises that will be legally binding on you. Thus, it is extremely important that you carefully review any contract before you sign it.

It is highly recommended you consult your personal attorney before signing any contract. The ADA also offers an important resource for ADA members – the ADA Contract Analysis Service. Prior to signing a proposed contract, member dentists may submit a dental provider contract with a third-party payer or a dental management service organization to their state or local dental society who will forward it to the Service for a free analysis. The service provides a plain language explanation of proposed contract terms for each agreement analyzed. The service does not provide legal advice or recommend whether a contract should or should not be signed.

You have the right to negotiate the terms of a participating dentist agreement; however, the plan also has contractual rights that may affect your rights. It certainly doesn't hurt to ask if you have concerns with specific clauses in the participating dentist agreement.

Many times, if a dentist has contracted with a third-party payer, he or she may have agreed to abide by the carrier's processing policies, which may or may not appear in the contract itself. The processing policies of many carriers are published on their websites. Dentists should make it a point to understand the policies typically applied by payers.

And don't forget to ask for the plan's current dentist billing manual and be sure you understand how the plan processes the procedures that you most frequently perform.

Remember not to focus only on the contract itself – after all, you are making a business decision and data is very important. Your practice management software typically has reporting tools that many dentists may not be aware of and do not utilize to their own advantage. It may be a good time to call your software vendor to learn how to generate reports that will help you better understand your own practice metrics.

It is also important for dental offices to understand payer processing policies before treatment is started so that these policies can be adequately explained to patients. Patients often rely on their dentists and office staff to decode their dental benefits for them and the dentist-patient relationship can be affected by payer policies.

Treatment plans should cater to the needs of the patient rather than what is covered by the benefit plan. Always remember to "code for what you do and do what you coded for." Although the payer may bundle codes for the purpose of benefit determination, the patient record should always accurately describe the services that the patient received. You always have the right to appeal the claim decision, especially in instances where the payer has made a judgment regarding the medical necessity of a treatment you provided your patient.

Helping You After You Sign the Contract

Sometimes legislation may be the best approach to dealing with issues related to dental benefit plans. The ADA's Washington, DC office has many efforts underway to address dental benefit issues through legislative remedies.

Examples of current efforts include:

1. Non-Covered Services
2. Assignment of Benefits
3. Coordination of Benefits
4. Flexible Spending Accounts

Non-Covered Services

A key concern reported to ADA by dental offices has been carriers use of requiring dentists to charge patients the plan's maximum allowable fee for services not covered by the dental plan. The ADA is working closely with its state partners and has helped implement legislation in 38 states that prohibits dental plans from forcing dentists to accept the plan's maximum allowable fee for a non-covered procedure.

Bundling and Downcoding

Examples of provisions in the signed contract that limit reimbursement include bundling and downcoding, which has resulted in many dental offices calling the ADA asking for guidance. If the payer has applied some of these limitations and they are in accordance with the contract with which the dentist agreed, the dentist may be bound to the policies set forth by the payer.

The ADA defines bundling of procedures as the systematic combining of distinct dental procedure codes by third-party payers that results in a reduced benefit for the patient/beneficiary.

Downcoding is a practice of third-party payers in which the benefit code has been changed to a less complex or lower cost procedure than was reported, except where delineated in contract agreements.

Let's look at an example of downcoding. A 13-year-old patient with adult dentition is treated and the dentist has rendered a **D0120 periodic oral evaluation** and **D1110 prophylaxis – adult**.

The payer rejected the claim for D1110 and returned an explanation of benefits (EOB) statement indicating the correct code is D1120 prophylaxis – child, as this is the correct code because the dental benefit plan defines a patient under age 15 as a child, no matter what dentition is present. This is worth an appeal because the message implies that that the dentist miscoded the claim, which is not true.

An appeal could be avoided if the EOB acknowledged that the reimbursement was based on benefit plan design. It is important to note that appealing a claim may not always result in greater reimbursement but could simply help prevent misperceptions by the patient.

In this scenario, the claim was not adjudicated correctly as the payer ignored the D1110 descriptor and asked the dentist to report the wrong procedure code. The only proper action for the dentist is to code for what you do.

Now let's look at an example of bundling. The dentist provided a **D0120 periodic oral evaluation**, **D1120 prophylaxis – child** and **D1208 topical application of fluoride – excluding varnish** to a 6 year old patient. The payer rejected the claim and the EOB implied that all three procedures were part of the same CDT Code. Once again, this is a situation that should be appealed to correct the language within the EOB statement.

In this case, the payer ignored the nomenclatures and descriptors of these discrete codes and redefined procedure code D0120. A third-party payer is supposed to use the code number, its nomenclature and its descriptor as written.

It is not acceptable when a payer says the procedure reported with D0120 includes other procedures, in this instance – D1120 and D1208 – that are appropriately reported separately on the claim form. In this particular example the payer may even be in violation of its CDT Code license.

It is okay when a payer benefits procedures in combination with others as part of its payment policies, but the payer cannot claim that discrete procedures are actually part of other procedures.

Refund Requests and Overpayments

Some contracts may have clauses that contractually bind you to refund any overpayments. Many times when a third-party payer mistakenly pays a dentist, the payer will request a refund of the overpaid amount. In some cases, refund requests have been sent to dentists more than two years after the payment was made and the patient may no longer be a patient of record. In most instances, the overpaid amount is deducted from future benefits paid to the dentist. In some cases, overpayments made to other dentists for the same patient may be deducted from future benefit payments to the current treating dentist. Many members and the ADA question the fairness of this practice.

Several states have enacted legislation that restricts how far back a carrier can ask for a refund and a period of one year seems to be the most common. Ensuring you understand these clauses is of the utmost importance before signing a participating dentist agreement with a third-party payer.

Removal From Network Lists

If a dentist wants to terminate an agreement, there is usually a range of 30 to 90 days before a termination will take effect. Dental offices have reported that although a contract with a third-party payer was terminated previously, the carrier did not update its website with correct information. Patients were under the false impression that the dentist was still contracted with the plan and were expecting the carrier's discounted fees, not the dentist's full fees.

This can cause major problems for the patient and the dental office and may even interfere with the dentist-patient relationship. As a best practice, at the time of cancellation dentists should submit in writing, to the carrier (sent via certified mail) a request specifically to remove their names from any participating dentist list.

Dentists should follow up with carriers who fail to remove their name in a timely manner. Please call the ADA for assistance if your name has not been removed from the plan's website after the termination date.

What Fee Should I Submit?

A question frequently asked by dental offices is what fee to report on the claim form: the discounted fee or the dentist's full fee? Irrespective of whether you are contracted or not contracted, the ADA recommends that dentists should always submit their full fee to carriers. The carriers will be certain to only allow the agreed upon fees for payment.

Helping the Non-Contracted Dentist

Many dental carriers will not honor assignment of benefits to non-contracted dentists. These plans claim that assignment of benefits is a contracted dentist benefit. The good news is that 22 states have passed legislation requiring that assignment of benefits be honored. These laws generally apply only to fully insured plans which are governed by state insurance statutes and approximately 52% of patients with a dental benefit have a plan that is insured and subject to state laws. If your state has not passed assignment of benefits legislation, it is recommended you talk to your state dental society about doing so.

Helping All Dentists

Payment Delay and Lost Submissions

One of the biggest complaints concerning third-party claim payment is lost claim forms and radiographs. Many dentists report sending in claim forms or radiographs several times before the dental plan will acknowledge receipt. Often radiographs are submitted with the claim, but the dentist will receive an EOB requesting the radiographs.

In some instances, the method by which claims are submitted increases the possibility of loss. Attachments that are not firmly affixed to a claim form can get separated when the mail is opened; this is especially true when multiple claims are submitted in one envelope. If radiographs are not labeled and get detached from claim forms, they may not be able to be matched back to the appropriate claim form. Privacy and security standards require that personal medical information be protected so unmatched attachments would most likely be destroyed.

When a payer does not require a radiograph for a claim, the process established by that payer may require that the radiograph be removed and returned or destroyed. If a subsequent issue moves the claim from auto-adjudication to a manual review, a radiograph may be requested at that time.

Submitting electronic claims and the appropriate attachments to them is the best way to avoid the loss of claims, radiographs and other attachments.

There is no uniformity within the payer community regarding submission of radiographs, partly due to different business structures within the industry. Some companies would prefer that no radiographs be sent unless requested. Others want to see images at the time specific procedure codes are reported.

Top Procedure Denials

- **Periodontal scaling and root planing (D4341, D4342) and periodontal maintenance (D4910)**

  Scaling and root planing (SRP) denials are one of the most reported concerns to the ADA. Dentists believe that submitted radiographs show bone loss substantial enough to warrant coverage for SRP and have reported that dentist consultants working for payers deny these claims indicating there is no radiographic evidence of bone loss. Upon appeal some of these claims have been paid.

  Dentists and their staff may not always understand what appears to be inconsistent SRP claim adjudication as payer adjudication policies vary substantially. One plan may require at least 4mm pocket depth while another may have different depth criteria. Many plans will require radiographic evidence of bone loss before paying an SRP claim. Some payers may not benefit more than two quadrants of scaling and root planing performed on the same date of service.

  It is very difficult for a small dental office to be familiar with the various payer requirements for payment of SRP claims as it is typical for a dental office to have patients present with well over 100 different dental plans.

  A major concern of dental offices is that the denial language used on the EOB statement may lead the patient to think that the procedure was not necessary. Denial of benefits may not mean the SRP was unnecessary – it simply means the patient's clinical condition did not satisfy the benefit plan's threshold for reimbursement.

  In addition to radiographic evidence of bone loss, it is not uncommon for payers to request periodontal charting and a narrative description for SRP coverage consideration.

  Claim denials for D4910 periodontal maintenance occur because some carriers have limited benefits for D4910. Some plans reimburse only if periodontal maintenance was delivered within 2 to 12 months of scaling and root planing while others may require a 3-month wait after therapy. Some plans deny benefits unless 2 or more quadrants have received prior therapy; however, there are no such limitations in the CDT Code.

It is recommended that dental office staff determine how a patient's plan covers this procedure before delivery in order to better inform the patient of the coverage parameters so as to avoid any claim surprises. If known, tell patients in advance that plan provisions may not provide for reimbursement of D4910 for extended periods of time and that the patient may be responsible for the costs.

- **Crowns (D2710 – D2799) and core buildups (D2950)**

  The ADA receives many calls on crown and core buildup denials and there are myriad reasons for these denials. Some carriers use a policy for crowns that is along the lines of requiring that at least 50% of the incisal angle must need replacement due to decay or fracture. In addition, many carriers will deny crowns for a tooth with a poor prognosis and due to abrasion and attrition. Core buildups are typically covered once every 5 years if there is less than 50% tooth structure due to disease or fracture. Many payers will require documentation, including radiographs and a narrative description, for coverage consideration.

  The ADA has received calls from dental offices where carriers' EOBs have stated that only the crown should be reported as it includes the core buildup. In this example, the payer is incorrect per the CDT Code's perspective as the buildup procedure and crown procedure are separate and distinct from each other as not all crowns require a buildup.

  It is understood that the payer can make single reimbursement based on benefit plan design, and this should be made clear on the EOB statement sent to the patient. The dentist should be able to balance bill the patient; however, the ability to balance bill is subject to the participating dentist agreement, if any.

  To avoid post-treatment complaints, dental offices should help patients understand the clinical basis for treatment and should appeal the benefit decision if it is thought the claim has not been properly adjudicated.

Compliance Audits and Utilization Review

Many dental offices call the ADA when confronted with a compliance audit or with questions on utilization review. When a dentist is placed under utilization review, the office is often required to submit additional documentation for the procedures being questioned. These claims are then manually reviewed to determine the benefit.

Some carriers require that claims being reviewed be sent to a different address than where you would normally send claims. If you are being audited, please be sure to send audit documentation to the correct address provided by the dental plan. Otherwise it will slow down the processing of your claim submission.

When you are notified of being placed under review or are suddenly receiving requests for additional documentation, it is recommended you contact the dental plan's consultant or your provider relations manager to determine if a review is being undertaken and, if it is, why you were placed on utilization review and what it will take to get you off of the plan's utilization review.

The plan is obligated to disclose the results of your review. Please do not forget your right to appeal. You have the right to appeal the reasons why you have been placed on utilization review.

It is recommended you work with the plan to explain and justify potential differences in practice patterns, e.g., a dental office that caters to elderly patients may indeed have higher utilization patterns for bridges. This is something that could be explained and taken into consideration by the dental plan. Helping the dental plan understand the rationale for your recommended treatment plans can help significantly.

Remember to properly and accurately document your patient records to the very last detail, even if something appears obvious to you. It may be a good idea to submit pre-treatment estimates when you are under review, so as to minimize any surprises.

Over time if the payer is assured that treatment patterns are justified then the payer will remove the dentist from further review. However, in some instances the payer may choose to follow up with an in-office audit.

In the event of an in-office audit, plan representatives will personally visit your office to review patient files and records. The plan will request that a separate work area be set up for them to conduct the review and you will be asked in advance to have specific patient records available for review by plan representatives.

Auditors and plan representatives may look at claims as far back as state laws allow. Please note that in-office reviews can last one or more days depending on the number of records to be reviewed.

If you are contracted with the plan and have agreed to such audits, it is recommended that you read and familiarize yourself with your contract and the plan's policies before the audit begins.

We also encourage dentists to obtain a written description of the scope of the audit procedures. Consulting with your personal attorney so that you understand your rights and obligations in such a situation is also recommended.

It may be a good idea to talk with your plan representative about the following before the audit begins:

- Clinical review criteria
- Analytical methods
- Time periods for conducting reviews
- Qualifications of individuals conducting the review
- Confidentiality
- Disclosure of the process to insured's
- Access to review staff
- Appeals process for adverse determinations

A question we often receive is whether the dentist is allowed to disclose a patient's record to the plan in cases of an audit. The HIPAA Privacy Rule permits a dental practice to disclose such information in response to such a request if the dental plan has or had relationships with the individuals who are the subjects of the requested information. An important point to note is that for patients who have been beneficiaries of the plan in the past and are no longer deriving benefits from that plan, the payer's auditor can only look at the patient's records for the time the patient was part of the plan.

Individual patients have a right to request that disclosures not be made to a health or dental plan for services that the patient has paid for out of pocket and in full. A covered dental practice may not disclose information regarding patients who are not, and have never been beneficiaries of that plan, even if a participating dentist agreement requires it. Disclosing the information may be in violation of HIPAA.

When a patient has paid for a service in full and asks the practice not to disclose the service to the plan, the dental practice must comply with that request. As a best practice, a notice of privacy practices (NPP) should be given to individuals at their first visit. The NPP should contain information about the patient's rights with regards to HIPAA and how the patient may request restrictions on disclosures of information. Your practice must also have procedures for your staff to flag such requests in the event of such a request coming from a patient, written or otherwise.

Resources

- The Center for Professional Success website offers a plethora of information on dental benefits at *ADA.org/dentalbenefits*.
- Information on the Code on Dental Procedures and Nomenclature (CDT Code), as well as the review and revision process, is available at *ADA.org/cdt*.
- *Why Doesn't My Insurance Pay for This?* (W265) is a brochure designed to help patients understand dental benefit plans by explaining why some procedures are not covered and it describes annual maximums, least expensive alternative treatment clauses, pre-existing conditions, exclusions and more. Available at *ADAcatalog.org*.
- *What Every Dentist Should Know Before Signing a Dental Provider Contract* is a publication that answers common questions dentists may wish to consider before signing a dental contract with third-party payers. Available at *www.ADA.org/thirdpartycontract*.
- *CDT 2019: Dental Procedure Codes* (J019) is the most up-to-date coding resource on the market will help you document codes for dental procedures quickly and accurately. This book not only helps fill documentation gaps, but can help reduce rejected dental claims. Available at *ADAcatalog.org*.
- *CDT 2019 Coding Companion* (J449) trains staff to code accurately and efficiently with key coding concepts, various scenarios and FAQs. Available at *ADAcatalog.org*.
- *Third-Party Concerns* is a series of articles published in ADA News on third-party problems reported by dental offices. Available at *success.ADA.org/en/dental-benefits/member-support-on-third-party-issues.*
- *Decoding Dental Benefits* is a series of ADA News articles seeks to educate dentists so informed decisions on dental plan participation can be made. Available at *success.ADA.org/en/dental-benefits/decoding-dental-benefits-series.*
- *Responding to Claim Rejections* is a publication that educates dentists and dental offices on the proper way to handle and respond to claim rejections from third-party payers. Available at *ADAcatalog.org/cpspdf.aspx?assets=2187&day=b1mygiq+JiA.*

- *Dental Benefit Series Videos* are short video tutorials, created by the ADA Center for Dental Benefits, Coding and Quality, are designed to help dental professionals understand a key issue in dentistry: how third-party programs interface with dental offices. Available at ***success.ada.org/en/dental-benefits/dental-benefit-videos?utm_source=promospots&utm_content=dentalbenefitslp&utm_medium=fb&utm_campaign=easy.***

- Dental Benefit Webinars are a series of recorded webinars on various dental benefit topics ***success.ada.org/en/dental-benefits/dental-benefit-webinars?utm_source=promospots&utm_content=dentalbenefitslp&utm_medium=fb&utm_campaign=easy***.

- *The ADA Practical Guide to Dental Letters* (J053) contains sample letters addressing third-party issues, including UCR and EOB language which may be customized to send to patients' employers and third-party payers as appropriate. Available at ***ADAcatalog.org***.

- ADA Contract Analysis Service (ADA members only) is available at ***ADA.org/en/member-center/member-benefits/legal-resources/contract-analysis-service.***

Section 3.
Appendices

Appendix 1: CDT Code to ICD (Diagnosis) Code Cross-Walk

CDT Code(s)	
D0120	periodic oral evaluation – established patient
D0140	limited oral evaluation – problem focused
D0150	comprehensive oral evaluation – new or established patient
D0210	intraoral – complete series of radiographic images
D0220	intraoral – periapical first radiographic image
D0230	intraoral – periapical each additional radiographic image
D0251	extra-oral posterior dental radiographic image
D0272	bitewings – two radiographic images
D0274	bitewings – four radiographic images
D0330	panoramic radiographic image
D0999	unspecified diagnostic procedure, by report
Suggested ICD-10-CM Diagnosis Code(s)	
Z01.20	Encounter for dental examination and cleaning without abnormal findings
Z01.21	Encounter for dental examination and cleaning with abnormal findings
Z13.84	encounter screening for dental disorders

CDT Code(s)	
D1110	prophylaxis – adult
D1120	prophylaxis – child
Suggested ICD-10-CM Diagnosis Code(s)	
E11.9	Type 2 diabetes mellitus without complications
K03.6	Deposits [accretions] on teeth
K05.1	Chronic gingivitis
K05.10	Chronic gingivitis, plaque induced
K05.30	Chronic periodontitis
Z33.1	Pregnant state, incidental
Z72.0	Tobacco Use

CDT Code(s)	
D1206	topical application of fluoride varnish
D1208	topical application of fluoride, excluding varnish
Suggested ICD-10-CM Diagnosis Code(s)	
K02.3	Arrested dental caries
K02.61	Dental caries on smooth surface limited to enamel
K02.7	Dental root caries
K03.1	Abrasion of teeth
K03.2	Erosion of teeth
M35.00	Sicca syndrome*, unspecified

** also known as Sjögren's Syndrome*

CDT Code(s)	
D1330	oral hygiene instructions
Suggested ICD-10-CM Diagnosis Code(s)	
E11.9	Type 2 diabetes mellitus without complications
K02.3	Arrested dental caries
K02.52	Dental caries on pit and fissure surface penetrating into dentin
K02.61	Dental caries limited to enamel
K02.62	Dental caries on smooth surface penetrating into dentine
K02.7	Dental root caries
K02.9	Dental caries, unspecified
K03.2	Erosion of teeth
K03.6	Deposits [accretions] on teeth
K05.00	Acute gingivitis, plaque induced
K05.01	Acute gingivitis, non-plaque induced
K05.10	Chronic gingivitis, plaque induced
K05.30	Chronic periodontitis, unspecified
K05.5	Other periodontal diseases
M35.00	Sicca syndrome*, unspecified
Z33.1	Pregnant state, incidental
Z72.0	Tobacco use

** also known as Sjögren's Syndrome*

CDT Code(s)	
D1351	sealant – per tooth
D1354	interim caries arresting medicament application – per tooth
D2990	resin infiltration of incipient smooth surface lesions
Suggested ICD-10-CM Diagnosis Code(s)	
K02.51	Dental caries on pit and fissure surface limited to enamel
K02.61	Dental caries on smooth surface limited to enamel
M35.00	Sicca syndrome*, unspecified

** also known as Sjögren's Syndrome*

CDT Code(s)	
D1352	preventive resin restoration
Suggested ICD-10-CM Diagnosis Code(s)	
K02.51	Dental caries on pit and fissure surface limited to enamel

CDT Code(s)	
D2140	amalgam – one surface; primary or permanent
D2150	amalgam – two surfaces; primary or permanent
D2160	amalgam – three surfaces; primary or permanent
D2161	amalgam – four or more surfaces; primary or permanent
Suggested ICD-10-CM Diagnosis Code(s)	
K02.51	Dental caries on pit and fissure surface limited to enamel
K02.52	Dental caries on pit and fissure surface penetrating into dentin
K02.61	Dental caries on smooth surface limited to enamel
K02.62	Dental caries on smooth surface penetrating into dentin
K03.81	Cracked tooth
S02.5XXA	Fracture of tooth (traumatic), initial encounter for closed fracture

CDT Code(s)	
D2330	resin-based composite – one surface; anterior
D2331	resin-based composite – two surfaces; anterior
D2332	resin-based composite – three surfaces; anterior
D2335	resin-based composite – four or more surfaces or involving incisal angle (anterior)
Suggested ICD-10-CM Diagnosis Code(s)	
K00.2	Abnormalities of size and form of teeth
K02.51	Dental caries on pit and fissure surface limited to enamel
K02.52	Dental caries on pit and fissure surface penetrating into dentin
K02.61	Dental caries on smooth surface limited to enamel
K02.62	Dental caries on smooth surface penetrating into dentin
K03.1	Abrasion of teeth
K03.2	Erosion of teeth
K03.81	Cracked tooth
S02.5XXA	Fracture of tooth (traumatic), initial encounter for closed fracture

CDT Code(s)	
D2391	resin-based composite – one surface; posterior
D2392	resin-based composite – two surfaces; posterior
D2393	resin-based composite – three surfaces; posterior
D2394	resin-based composite – four or more surfaces; posterior
Suggested ICD-10-CM Diagnosis Code(s)	
K02.51	Dental caries on pit and fissure surface limited to enamel
K02.52	Dental caries on pit and fissure surface penetrating into dentin
K02.61	Dental caries on smooth surface limited to enamel
K02.62	Dental caries on smooth surface penetrating into dentin
K02.7	Dental root caries
K03.1	Abrasion of teeth
K03.2	Erosion of teeth
K03.81	Cracked tooth
S02.5XXA	Fracture of tooth (traumatic), initial encounter for closed fracture

CDT Code(s)	
D2740	crown – porcelain/ceramic
D2750	crown – porcelain fused to high noble metal
D2751	crown – porcelain fused to predominantly base metal
D2752	crown – porcelain fused to noble metal
D2790	crown – full cast high noble metal
D2792	crown – full cast noble metal
D2950	core buildup, including any pins when required
D2951	pin retention – per tooth; in addition to restoration
D2952	post and core in addition to crown; indirectly fabricated
D2954	prefabricated post and core in addition to crown
Suggested ICD-10-CM Diagnosis Code(s)	
K00.2	Abnormalities of size and form of teeth
K02.52	Dental caries on pit and fissure surface penetrating into dentin
K02.53	Dental caries on pit and fissure surface penetrating into pulp
K02.62	Dental caries on smooth surface penetrating into dentin
K02.63	Dental caries on smooth surface penetrating into pulp
S02.5XXA	Fracture of tooth (traumatic), initial encounter for closed fracture

CDT Code(s)	
D2930	prefabricated stainless steel crown – primary tooth
Suggested ICD-10-CM Diagnosis Code(s)	
K00.2	Abnormalities of size and form of teeth
K02.52	Dental caries on pit and fissure surface penetrating into dentine
K02.53	Dental caries on pit and fissure surface penetrating into pulp
K02.62	Dental caries on smooth surface penetrating into dentine
K02.63	Dental caries on smooth surface penetrating into pulp
S02.5XXA	Fracture of tooth (traumatic), initial encounter for closed fracture

CDT Code(s)	
D2940	protective restoration
Suggested ICD-10-CM Diagnosis Code(s)	
K02.9	Dental caries, unspecified
S02.5XXA	Fracture of tooth (traumatic), initial encounter for closed fracture

CDT Code(s)	
D3110	pulp cap – direct (excluding final restoration)
D3120	pulp cap – indirect (excluding final restoration)
Suggested ICD-10-CM Diagnosis Code(s)	
K02.52	Dental caries on pit and fissure surface penetrating into dentin
K02.53	Dental caries on pit and fissure surface penetrating into pulp
K02.62	Dental caries on smooth surface penetrating into dentin
K02.63	Dental caries on smooth surface penetrating into pulp
K04.0	Pulpitis
S02.5XXA	Fracture of tooth (traumatic), initial encounter for closed fracture

CDT Code(s)	
D3220	therapeutic pulpotomy (excluding final restoration) – removal of pulp coronal to the dentinocemental junction and application of medicament
D3310	endodontic therapy; anterior tooth (excluding final restoration)
D3320	endodontic therapy; premolar tooth (excluding final restoration)
D3330	endodontic therapy; molar tooth (excluding final restoration)
Suggested ICD-10-CM Diagnosis Code(s)	
K02.53	Dental caries on pit and fissure surface penetrating into pulp
K02.63	Dental caries on smooth surface penetrating into pulp
K03.81	Cracked tooth
K03.89	Other specified diseases of hard tissues of teeth
K04.0	Pulpitis
K04.1	Necrosis of pulp
K04.5	Chronic apical periodontitis
K04.6	Periapical abscess with sinus
K04.7	Periapical abscess without sinus
K04.8	Radicular cyst
K04.90	Unspecified diseases of pulp and periapical tissues
K04.99	Other diseases of pulp and periapical tissues
K05.5	Other periodontal diseases
K08.8	Other specified disorders of teeth and supporting structures
S02.5XXA	Fracture of tooth (traumatic), initial encounter for closed fracture

CDT Code(s)	
D3346	retreatment of previous root canal therapy – anterior
D3347	retreatment of previous root canal therapy – premolar
D3348	retreatment of previous root canal therapy – molar
Suggested ICD-10-CM Diagnosis Code(s)	
K08.59	Other unsatisfactory restoration of tooth
M27.5	Periradicular pathology associated with previous endodontic treatment

CDT Code(s)	
D4210	gingivectomy or gingivoplasty – four or more contiguous teeth or tooth bounded spaces per quadrant
D4211	gingivectomy or gingivoplasty – one to three contiguous teeth or tooth bounded spaces per quadrant
Suggested ICD-10-CM Diagnosis Code(s)	
K05.30	Chronic periodontitis, unspecified
K05.31	Chronic periodontitis, localized
K05.32	Chronic periodontitis, generalized
K06.1	Gingival enlargement

CDT Code(s)	
D4249	clinical crown lengthening – hard tissue
Suggested ICD-10-CM Diagnosis Code(s)	
K02.9	Dental caries, unspecified
K03.81	Cracked tooth
K05.5	Other periodontal diseases
S02.5XXA	Fracture of tooth (traumatic), initial encounter for closed fracture

CDT Code(s)	
D4260	osseous surgery (including elevation of a full thickness flap and closure) – four or more contiguous teeth or tooth bounded spaces per quadrant
D4261	osseous surgery (including elevation of a full thickness flap and closure) – one to three contiguous teeth or tooth bounded spaces per quadrant
D4263	bone replacement graft – retained natural tooth – first site in quadrant
D4264	bone replacement graft – retained natural tooth – each additional site in quadrant
Suggested ICD-10-CM Diagnosis Code(s)	
K05.21	Aggressive periodontitis, localized
K05.22	Aggressive periodontitis, generalized
K05.30	Chronic periodontitis
K05.31	Chronic periodontitis, localized
K05.32	Chronic periodontitis, generalized
K05.6	Periodontal disease, unspecified
K08.20	Unspecified atrophy of edentulous alveolar ridge
K08.21	Minimal atrophy of the mandible
K08.22	Moderate atrophy of the mandible
K08.23	Severe atrophy of the mandible
K08.24	Minimal atrophy of the maxilla
K08.25	Moderate atrophy of the maxilla
K08.26	Severe atrophy of the maxilla

CDT Code(s)	
D4270	pedicle soft tissue graft procedure
D4273	autogenous connective tissue graft procedure (including donor and recipient surgical sites) first tooth, implant or edentulous tooth position in graft
D4275	non-autogenous connective tissue graft (including recipient site and donor material) first tooth, implant, or edentulous tooth position in graft
D4276	combined connective tissue and double pedicle graft, per tooth
D4277	free soft tissue graft procedure (including recipient and donor surgical sites) first tooth, implant or edentulous tooth position in graft
D4278	free soft tissue graft procedure (including recipient and donor surgical sites) each additional contiguous tooth, implant or edentulous tooth position in same graft site
D4283	autogenous connective tissue graft procedure (including donor and recipient surgical sites) – each additional contiguous tooth, implant or edentulous tooth position in same graft site
D4285	non- autogenous connective tissue graft procedure (including recipient surgical site and donor material) – each additional contiguous tooth, implant or edentulous tooth position in same graft site
Suggested ICD-10-CM Diagnosis Code(s)	
K06.0	Gingival recession

CDT Code(s)	
D4341	periodontal scaling and root planing – four or more teeth per quadrant
D4342	periodontal scaling and root planing – one to three teeth per quadrant
D4346	scaling in the presence of generalized moderate or severe gingival inflammation – full mouth after oral evaluation
D4910	periodontal maintenance
D6081	scaling and debridement in the presence of inflammation or mucositis of a single implant, including cleaning of the implant surfaces, without flap entry and closure
Suggested ICD-10-CM Diagnosis Code(s)	
A69.1	Other Vincent's infections
E11.9	Type 2 diabetes mellitus without complications
K03.6	Deposits [accretions] on teeth
K05.20	Aggressive periodontitis, unspecified
K05.21	Aggressive periodontitis, localized
K05.22	Aggressive periodontitis, generalized
K05.30	Chronic periodontitis, unspecified
K05.31	Chronic periodontitis, localized
K05.32	Chronic periodontitis, generalized
K05.5	Other periodontal diseases
K05.6	Periodontal disease, unspecified
K06.1	Gingival enlargement
Z33.1	Pregnant state, incidental
Z72.0	Tobacco Use
Z87.891	Personal history of nicotine dependence

CDT Code(s)	
D4355	full mouth debridement to enable a comprehensive oral evaluation and diagnosis on a subsequent visit
Suggested ICD-10-CM Diagnosis Code(s)	
K03.6	Deposits [accretions] on teeth
Z72.0	Tobacco Use
Z87.891	Personal history of nicotine dependence

CDT Code(s)	
D5110	complete denture – maxillary
D5120	complete denture – mandibular
Suggested ICD-10-CM Diagnosis Code(s)	
K08.1	Complete loss of teeth

CDT Code(s)	
D5211	maxillary partial denture – resin base (including any conventional clasps, rests, and teeth)
D5212	mandibular partial denture - resin base (including retentive/clasping materials, rests, and teeth)
D5213	maxillary partial denture – cast metal framework with resin denture bases (including any conventional clasps; rests and teeth)
D5214	mandibular partial denture – cast metal framework with resin denture bases (including any conventional clasps; rests and teeth)
D6010	surgical placement of implant body: endosteal implant
D6056	prefabricated abutment – includes modification and placement
D6057	custom fabricated abutment – includes placement
D6059	abutment supported porcelain fused to metal crown (high noble metal)
D6240	pontic – porcelain fused to high noble metal
D6750	retainer crown – porcelain fused to high noble metal
D6752	retainer crown – porcelain fused to noble metal
Suggested ICD-10-CM Diagnosis Code(s)	
K00.00	Anodontia
K08.409	Partial loss of teeth, unspecified cause, unspecified class
K08.419	Partial loss of teeth due to trauma, unspecified class
K08.429	Partial loss of teeth due to periodontal diseases, unspecified class
K08.439	Partial loss of teeth due to caries, unspecified class

CDT Code(s)	
D7111	extraction; coronal remnants – primary tooth
D7250	removal of residual tooth roots (cutting procedure)
Suggested ICD-10-CM Diagnosis Code(s) – ICD-10-CM	
K03.9	Disease of hard tissues of teeth, unspecified

CDT Code(s)	
D7140	extraction; erupted tooth or exposed root (elevation and/or forceps removal)
D7210	extraction, erupted tooth requiring removal of bone and/or sectioning of tooth, and including elevation of mucoperiosteal flap if indicated
Suggested ICD-10-CM Diagnosis Code(s)	
K02.53	Dental caries on pit and fissure surface penetrating into pulp
K02.63	Dental caries on smooth surface penetrating into pulp
K04.0	Pulpitis
K04.1	Necrosis of the pulp
K04.5	Chronic apical periodontitis
K04.6	Periapical abscess with sinus
K04.7	Periapical abscess without sinus
K04.8	Radicular cyst
K05.21	Aggressive periodontitis, localized
K05.3	Chronic periodontitis
K08.439	Partial loss of teeth due to caries, unspecified class
K09.0	Developmental odontogenic cysts
L02.91	Cutaneous abscess, unspecified
L03.90	Cellulitis, unspecified
L03.91	Acute lymphangitis, unspecified
R44.8	Other symptoms and signs involving general sensations and perceptions
R44.9	Unspecified symptoms and signs involving general sensations and perceptions
R69	Illness, unspecified
S02.5XXA	Fracture of tooth (traumatic), initial encounter for closed fracture
S02.5XXB	Fracture of tooth (traumatic), initial encounter for open fracture
S03.2XXA	Dislocation of tooth, initial encounter

CDT Code(s)	
D7220	removal of impacted tooth – soft tissue
D7230	removal of impacted tooth – partially bony
D7240	removal of impacted tooth – completely bony
Suggested ICD-10-CM Diagnosis Code(s)	
K00.1	Supernumerary teeth
K00.6	Disturbances in tooth eruption
K01.0	Embedded teeth
K01.1	Impacted teeth
K09.0	Developmental odontogenic cysts

CDT Code(s)	
D7953	bone replacement graft for ridge preservation – per site
Suggested ICD-10-CM Diagnosis Code(s)	
K02.53	Dental caries on pit and fissure surface penetrating into pulp
K02.63	Dental caries on smooth surface penetrating into pulp
K04.0	Pulpitis
K04.1	Necrosis of pulp
K04.5	Chronic apical periodontitis
K04.6	Periapical abscess with sinus
K04.7	Periapical abscess without sinus
K04.8	Radicular cyst
K05.21	Aggressive periodontitis, localized
K05.30	Chronic periodontitis, unspecified
K05.31	Chronic periodontitis, localized
K05.32	Chronic periodontitis, generalized
K09.0	Developmental odontogenic cysts
S02.5XXA	Fracture of tooth (traumatic), initial encounter for closed fracture
S02.5XXB	Fracture of tooth (traumatic), initial encounter for open fracture
S03.2XXA	Dislocation of tooth, initial encounter

CDT Code(s)	
D8080	comprehensive orthodontic treatment of the adolescent dentition
Suggested ICD-10-CM Diagnosis Code(s)	
K00.0	Anodontia
K00.6	Disturbances in tooth eruption
K08.8	Other specified disorders of teeth and supporting structures
M26.212	Malocclusion, Angle's class II
M26.213	Malocclusion, Angle's class III
M26.24	Reverse articulation
M26.29	Other anomalies of dental arch relationship
M26.30	Unspecified anomaly of tooth position of fully erupted tooth or teeth
M26.31	Crowding of fully erupted teeth
M26.35	Rotation of fully erupted tooth or teeth
M26.39	Other anomalies of tooth position of fully erupted tooth or teeth
M26.4	Malocclusion, unspecified
M26.81	Anterior soft tissue impingement
M26.82	Posterior soft tissue impingement
M26.89	Other dentofacial anomalies
Q67.4	Other congenital deformities of skull, face, and jaw

CDT Code(s)	
D9110	palliative (emergency) treatment of dental pain – minor procedure
Suggested ICD-10-CM Diagnosis Code(s)	
K02.53	Dental caries on pit and fissure surface penetrating into pulp
K02.63	Dental caries on smooth surface penetrating into pulp
K04.0	Pulpitis
K04.6	Periapical abscess with sinus
K04.7	Periapical abscess without sinus
M26.60	Temporomandibular joint disorder, unspecified
M26.69	Other specified disorders of temporomandibular joint

CDT Code(s)	
D9230	inhalation of nitrous oxide/anxiolysis, analgesia
Suggested ICD-10-CM Diagnosis Code(s)	
F41.9	Anxiety disorder, unspecified

CDT Code(s)	
D9910	application of desensitizing medicament
Suggested ICD-10-CM Diagnosis Code(s)	
K03.0	Excessive attrition of teeth
K03.1	Abrasion of teeth
K03.2	Erosion of teeth

CDT Code(s)	
D9944	occlusal guard – hard appliance, full arch
D9945	occlusal guard – soft appliance, full arch
D9946	occlusal guard – hard appliance, partial arch
Suggested ICD-10-CM Diagnosis Code(s)	
F59	Unspecified behavioral syndromes associated with physiological disturbances and physical factors
K03.0	Excessive attrition of teeth
M26.60	Temporomandibular joint disorder, unspecified
M26.69	Other specified disorders of temporomandibular joint
M26.89	Other dentofacial anomalies

CDT Code(s)	
D9951	occlusal adjustment – limited
Suggested ICD-10-CM Diagnosis Code(s)	
K03.0	Excessive attrition of teeth
K03.81	Cracked Tooth
K04.0	Pulpitis
K06.0	Gingival recession
M26.60	Temporomandibular joint disorder, unspecified

Appendix 2:
A Guide to Reporting D4346

Some CDT Code changes, especially new codes, prompt a need for a coordinated educational message on the procedure and its reporting. The ADA, with support from organizations on the CMC and others in the dental community, develops and disseminates guidelines on these codes, which are available for everyone to read, download and share with others.

A Guide to Reporting D4346

The illustrated guidance to "D4346 scaling in presence of generalized moderate or severe gingival inflammation" discusses a code added in CDT 2017 that fills a procedure and reporting gap between a prophylaxis and a scaling and root planing (SRP). It is also available in PDF format online:

www.ada.org/publications/cdt/coding-guidance

ADA Guide to Reporting D4346

Developed by the ADA, this guide is published to educate dentists and others in the dental community on this scaling procedure and its approved code, first published in CDT 2017 and effective Jan 1, 2017

ADA Code of Ethics: Veracity

This is the foundation for the ADA's position –
"Code for what you do, and do what you coded for."

Section 5 of the *ADA Principles of Ethics and Code of Professional Conduct* is particularly applicable when determining the treatment plan and procedure coding.

SECTION 5 — Principle: Veracity ("truthfulness")

The dentist has a duty to communicate truthfully.

Code of Professional Conduct

5.A. Representation of Care. Dentists shall not represent the care being rendered to their patients in a false or misleading manner.

5.B. Representation of Fees. Dentists shall not represent the fees being charged for providing care in a false or misleading manner.

Advisory Opinions

5.B.5. Dental Procedures. A dentist who incorrectly describes on a third party claim form a dental procedure in order to receive a greater payment or reimbursement or incorrectly makes a non-covered procedure appear to be a covered procedure on such a claim form is engaged in making an unethical, false or misleading representation to such third party.

5.B.6. Unnecessary Services. A dentist who recommends and performs unnecessary dental services or procedures is engaged in unethical conduct. The dentist's ethical obligation in this matter applies regardless of the type of practice arrangement or contractual obligations in which he or she provides patient care.

Celebrating 150th year of the ADA Code of Ethics!

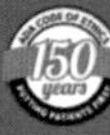

The full CDT Code entry –

D4346 scaling in presence of generalized moderate or severe gingival inflammation – full mouth, after oral evaluation

The removal of plaque, calculus and stains from supra- and sub-gingival tooth surfaces when there is generalized moderate or severe gingival inflammation in the absence of periodontitis. It is indicated for patients who have swollen, inflamed gingiva, generalized suprabony pockets, and moderate to severe bleeding on probing. Should not be reported in conjunction with prophylaxis, scaling and root planing, or debridement procedures.

ADA American Dental Association®
America's leading advocate for oral health

Visualizing the decision-making process: How a dentist decides whether or not the D4346 procedure is appropriate for a patient –

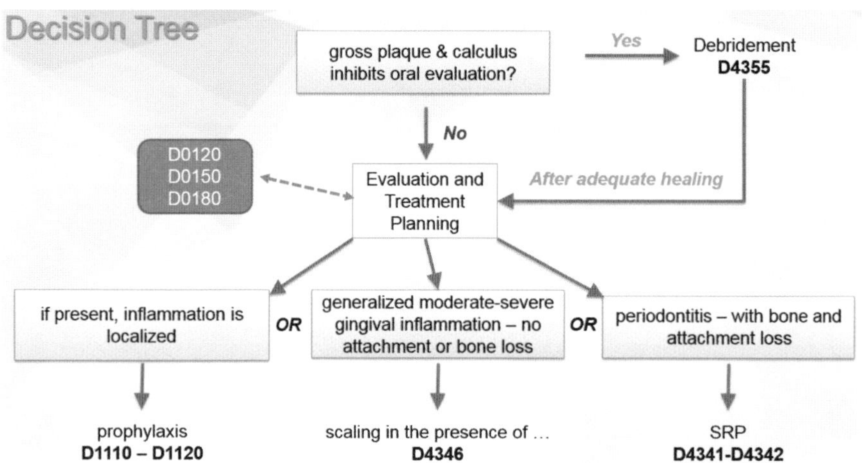

Questions and Answers

1. Why was a new "scaling" code added to the CDT Code?

a) Current CDT codes document procedures for patients with generally healthy periodontium, or patients with periodontal disease that has accompanying loss of attachment (e.g. periodontal pockets and bone loss).

- D1110 is primarily a preventive procedure, but can be therapeutic depending on the periodontium's overall health. It is applicable for patients with generally healthy periodontium where any deposits are removed to control irritational factors, and for patients with localized gingivitis to prevent further progression of the disease.
- Codes D4341 and D4342 are therapeutic procedures, and are indicated for patients who require scaling and root planing due to bone loss and subsequent loss of attachment. Instrumentation of the exposed root surface to remove deposits is an integral part of this procedure.
- There is no CDT Code available to report therapeutic treatment of patients with generalized moderate to severe gingival inflammation, with or without pseudo-pockets but exhibiting no bone loss – this is the gap filled by D4346.

b) Filling this gap will result in more accurate documentation and reporting by eliminating consideration of:

- D4999 as this code requires a narrative containing information that limits auto-adjudication
- "Undercoding" as a Prophylaxis procedure
- "Overcoding" as a Scaling and Root Planing procedure

ADA American Dental Association®
America's leading advocate for oral health

2. **Would the D4346 procedure be appropriate for a "hard prophy" where more time than usual is required to remove plaque, calculus and excessive staining from the tooth structures in order to control local irritational factors?**

   If the "hard prophy" is being defined strictly by the amount of time required to complete the procedure, then no D4346 is not appropriate. The D4346 procedure is applicable when there is generalized moderate or severe gingival inflammation in the absence of attachment loss. In other words, the procedure is based on the diagnosis rather than intensity of treatment required.

3. **How do you differentiate this new scaling procedure (D4346) from the current debridement procedure (D4355)?**

   D4355 is an enabler for comprehensive oral evaluation – i.e. it is performed before the subsequent comprehensive evaluation simply to remove gross deposits from the tooth surface. D4346 is a therapeutic service performed after evaluation and diagnosis of gingivitis to remove all deposits and allow tissue healing.

4. **What sort of oral evaluation is appropriate before delivery of D4346?**

   As with all therapeutic procedures, D4346 is performed after a periodic (D0120), comprehensive (D0150), or comprehensive periodontal (D0180) oral evaluation.

5. **May the oral evaluation and the D4346 procedure be performed on the same date of service?**

   Yes. There is nothing in either CDT code's nomenclature or descriptor that precludes their delivery and reporting on the same date of service.

6. **What is the clear and accepted definition of "...generalized moderate to severe gingival inflammation..." so that the D4346 procedure can be differentiated from prophylaxis procedures?**

   a) The AAP defines generalized chronic periodontitis[1] to be when 30% or more of the patient's teeth at one or more sites are involved, and it is reasonable to extend this definition to a patient with gingivitis.

      [1] *(J. Perio July 2015 American Academy of Periodontology Task Force Report on the Update to the 1999 Classification of Periodontal Diseases and Conditions [Original reference – Consensus Report: Chronic Periodontitis. 1999 International Workshop for a Classification of Periodontal Diseases and Conditions. Ann Periodontol 1999;4:38])*

   b) The Gingival Index of Lőe and Silness defines gingival inflammation as follows:

      0 = normal gingiva

      1 = mild inflammation- slight change in color and slight edema but no bleeding on probing

      2 = moderate inflammation- redness, edema, and glazing, bleeding on probing

      3 = severe inflammation- marked redness and edema, ulceration with tendency to spontaneous bleeding.

7. **What procedure is appropriate for patients with localized gingival inflammation (gingivitis)?**

   D1110 is applicable for patients with localized gingivitis to prevent further progression of the disease.

8. **What procedure is appropriate for a patient who has recession without pockets or inflammation (meaning the remaining periodontium is healthy), and no history of SRP – should I consider D1110, D4341/D4342 or D4346?**

   A prophylaxis procedure is appropriate and is documented with CDT code D0110. If there were pockets and inflammation an SRP (D4341/D4342) could be delivered. The D4346 procedure is not applicable since the patient does not present with gingival inflammation.

9. Is there a waiting period between completion of a D4346 and delivery of a prophylaxis as part of the patient's routine preventive regimen?

There is no set waiting period. D4346 is a therapeutic procedure to bring the patients periodontium back to health. Based on the patients' needs, the dentist is in the best position to determine when the patient can assume a regular preventive regimen that includes oral prophylaxis.

10. D4346 is a full mouth procedure; does this mean that it is completed in a single day?

This procedure is expected to be completed on a single date of service, but patient comfort and acceptance may require delivery over more than one visit. Should more than one day be required the date of completion is the date of service.

11. What dental professional would deliver the D4346 procedure?

As with all procedures documented with CDT codes, state laws regulating scope of practice determine which persons may deliver the service.

12. Is local anesthesia used when delivering D4346?

Patient needs and preferences, as well as the clinical state of the dentition, are factors that the dentist considers when determining the need for local anesthesia. State law determines who may deliver the anesthetic agent, which would be documented on the patient's record using the applicable CDT code.

13. What should be documented in the patient's record to support delivery of D4346?

a) Periodontal charting that records (pseudo) pocket depths and bleeding on probing. (Note: Pocket depth may be recorded without loss of attachment.)

b) Diagnostic images (type and frequency to be determined by the dentist) may be helpful to document the gingiva's condition (e.g., visualize localized v. generalized inflammation) for retention in the patient's chart.

14. Is D4346 a procedure followed by periodontal maintenance reported with D4910?

No. D4346 is performed in patients who do not exhibit any loss of attachment. D4910 is a procedure that includes site specific root planing as needed in patients who have been treated for attachment loss.

15. The procedure reported with CDT code – "D6081 scaling and debridement in the presence of inflammation or mucositis of a single implant, including cleaning of the implant surfaces, without flap" may be part of the treatment plan for a patient who also has moderate to severe gingival inflammation. Could D6081 and D4346 be delivered to the patient on the same date of service?

Yes. Both D6081 and D4346 may be delivered on the same date of service as there is nothing in either CDT code's nomenclature or descriptor that precludes concurrent delivery and reporting.

Please note, however, that D6081's descriptor does preclude delivery and reporting on the same date of service that either D1110 or D4910 are delivered.

ADA American Dental Association®
America's leading advocate for oral health

16. What do you mean by "Loss of attachment"?

This term is defined (*Stedman's Medical Dictionary for Dental Professionals; 1st Edition, 2007*) as: "Damage to the structures that support the tooth; results from periodontitis and is characterized by relocation of the junctional epithelium to the tooth root, destruction of the fibers of the gingiva, destruction of the periodontal ligament fibers, and loss of alveolar bone support from around the tooth." (see illustration). **Loss of attachment results from loss of bone.**

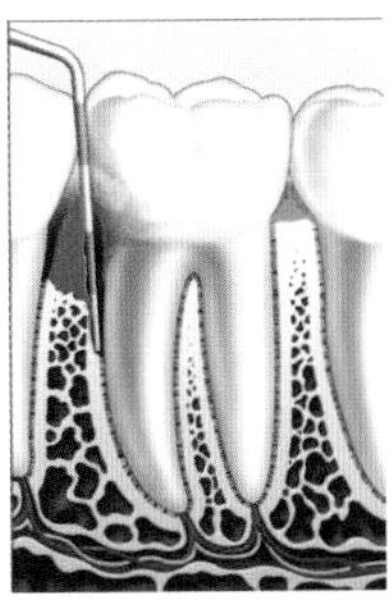

17. Why was the procedure for "scaling in the presence of...generalized gingival inflammation" assigned a code in the CDT Code's "D4xxx" (Periodontics) category rather than in "D1xxx (Preventive)?

The procedure is considered therapeutic for a patient in a diseased state, as noted by the following sentence in the D4346 descriptor – "It is indicated for patients who have swollen, inflamed gingiva, generalized suprabony pockets, and moderate to severe bleeding on probing." When a patient is diagnosed with generalized gingivitis following an oral evaluation this scaling procedure **treats** the generalized gingival inflammation and pseudopockets present.

18. Can a patient who received the D4346 scaling procedure then receive a D4341 (or D4342) scaling and root planing procedure?

There is no exclusionary language in the nomenclatures or descriptors of D4346, D4341 or D4342, as dentists recognize that periodontal disease may be progressive. The CDT Code fully supports documentation and reporting of procedures at any time the dentist determines they are necessary for the patient's oral health. This is a matter of clinical judgment by the treating dentist. Benefit design should not guide the clinical determination of procedure performed. For example:

[1] <u>Scenario 1</u>: A patient presents and after an oral evaluation the dentist determines that there is generalized moderate to severe gingival inflammation **without** attachment or bone loss. **The treatment plan based on this evaluation is delivery of D4346.** When completed the patient receives oral hygiene instruction that when followed would reduce the likelihood of continued or recurring inflammation.

On a later date the same patient presents, complaining of bleeding gums or at the next scheduled oral evaluation, the dentist notices that the patient now has periodontitis with attachment and bone loss. In this event a **new treatment plan** is prepared that includes scaling and root planing procedures (e.g., D4341 or D4342). For this recurrent episode of disease scaling (D4346) is not repeated prior to SRP because the patient has bone loss.

[2] <u>Scenario 2</u>: A patient presents and is diagnosed with localized or generalized **periodontitis** with evidence of bone loss. The treatment plan based on this evaluation is scaling and root planing (D4341 or D4342). Any subsequent treatment would be either periodontal maintenance (D4910) or repeating the SRP treatment. The D4346 procedure is not applicable as part of initial or subsequent treatment in this scenario because the patient exhibits bone loss, and "scaling" is an inherent component of the SRP procedure.

The following chart illustrates these and other clinical scenarios.

ADA American Dental Association®
America's leading advocate for oral health

Findings upon evaluation		Treatment rendered/ planned
Gingiva	**Attachment/Bone**	**Procedure Code**
Generally healthy, if present gingival inflammation is localized	Healthy - No attachment or bone loss	D1110
Generalized moderate to severe gingivitis	Healthy - No attachment or bone loss[1]	D4346 (No D1110)
Localized gingivitis	Localized bone loss[2]	D1110 + SRP as applicable (D4341, D4342) + other treatment as needed*
Generalized gingivitis	Localized or generalized bone loss[2]	D1110 + SRP as applicable (D4341, D4342) + other treatment as needed*

*Note: This guide does not address other treatments for periodontitis (e.g. osseous surgery, bone graft etc.) that may be planned to treat the disease.

19. If one quadrant of scaling and root planing is performed because there is bone loss only in that quadrant, can you report 4346 for the rest of the mouth on the same date of service?

According to the D4346 descriptor this procedure "...Should not be reported in conjuction with prophylaxis, *scaling and root planing* [emphasis added] or debridement procedures." In an exceptional situation the dentist could submit a claim for both services with an explanatory narrative. This would not necessarily result in reimbursement for the separate scaling procedure.

20. What would be an appropriate fee for the D4346 procedure – something between a prophylaxis fee and a scaling and root planing fee?

Each dentist who decides to deliver the D4346 procedure would set an appropriate fee, which may be adjusted with experience. One dentist might consider a value between a D1110 and a D4341, while another may not. This is each dentist's business decision.

There is no claim history for the D4346 procedure, or fee survey information. Dental benefit plan designers and administrators are in a similar situation regarding reimbursement amounts and frequency. It will likely be some time before aggregate fee or reimbursement information will be available.

21. Are there any frequency limitations on the scaling procedure?

Patient needs differ and the dentist's clinical evaluation determines when the D4346 procedure is indicated to maintain oral health. Dental benefit plans may, however, have coverage limitations or exclusions that may limit available reimbursements. It is important that the patient understand that not all procedures needed to maintain oral health or address dental disease are covered by dental benefit plans.

22. How often will a dental benefit plan provide coverage and reimbursement for the D4346 procedure?

The CDT Code provides a means to document and report services rendered. Reimbursement as with all codes is determined by provisions of the patient's dental benefits plan. The patients dental plan determines coverage and defines which services are covered as well as limitations and exclusions, which may vary, based on regulatory requirements and/ or the level of coverage.

It is likely that coverage limitations and reimbursement amounts will vary between dental benefit plans as such matters are often determined through actuarial experience. It is also likely that payers will take into account the rate of progression of periodontal disease when determining a frequency limitation to the D4346 and follow-up D4341/D4342 procedures. The best way to know is to ask the carrier (e.g., submit a pre-determination request).

23. If radiographs on the date of service are not required as part of the D4346 procedure, what about periodontal charting – considering both patient record-keeping and claim submission?

From the record keeping perspective the patient's record should contain necessary radiographs and charting within the last year to document the state of inflammation, pocketing and loss of atachment or bone. Photographs taken on the date of service are also helpful for visual documentation. Any patient who shows sign of disease should have an up to date chart and images in their record. The American Academy of Periodontology (AAP) recommends annual charting.

24. Patients with full mouth implant supported prostheses without any natural teeth have abutments and prostheses that need to be cleaned regularly. Because the D4346 CDT Code entry does not specify the type of tooth involved – natural or prosthetic – is it appropriate to use this code for such regular cleaning?

The D4346 procedure is applicable to natural teeth as it's descriptor describes the procedure as "…removal of plaque, calculus and stains from supra- and sub-gingival *tooth surfaces* [emphasis added]…" According to the D6080 nomenclature that procedure applies to implants.

Snapshot of differences between procedure codes

Attribute	Procedure			
Nomenclature	prophylaxis – adult; prophylaxis – child	scaling in the presence of generalized moderate or severe gingival inflammation – full mouth after oral evaluation	periodontal scaling and root planing – four or more *(or one to three)* teeth per quadrant	periodontal maintenance
CDT Code	D1110 D1120	D4346	D4341 D4342	D4910
Precursor Procedure(s)	oral evaluation	oral evaluation diagnostic image(s)	oral evaluation diagnostic image(s) including radiographs	active periodontal therapy (following SRP, Gingival Flap, or Osseous surgery)
Procedure features	scaling and polishing	sub-gingival (pseudo-pockets) scaling and polishing	sub-gingival (pockets with loss of attachments) scaling and polishing	scaling, polishing, and root planing (site specific)
Clinical condition	Localized gingival inflammation, if any	generalized moderate to severe gingival inflammation	periodontal disease including loss of attachment	ongoing therapy to treat periodontal disease

ADA American Dental Association®
America's leading advocate for oral health

Clinical Scenarios

1. Illustrations of situations where gross debridement may be applicable

D4355 full mouth debridement to enable a comprehensive evaluation and diagnosis on a subsequent visit

Full mouth debridement involves the preliminary removal of plaque and calculus that interferes with the ability of the dentist to perform a comprehensive oral evaluation. Not to be completed on the same day as D0150, D0160 or D0170.

Note the generalized nature of deposits. Periodontal probing and charting may be difficult in such a case, and debridement could facilitate the comprehensive oral evaluation.

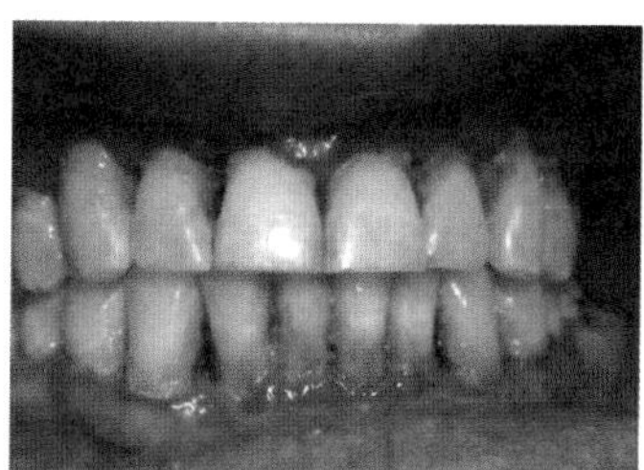

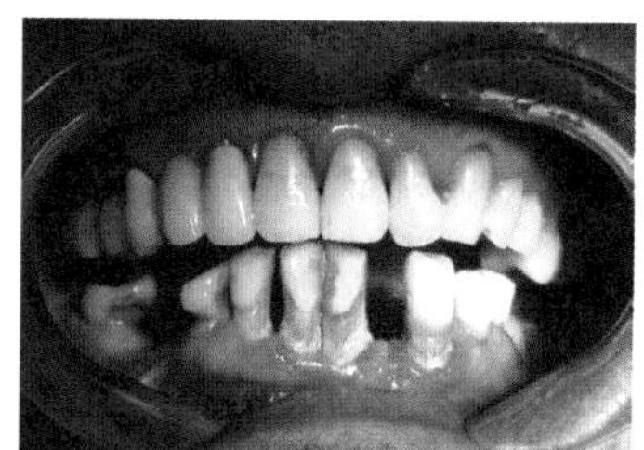

2. Illustrations of situations where oral prophylaxis may be applicable

D1110 prophylaxis – adult

Removal of plaque, calculus and stains from the tooth structures in the permanent and transitional dentition. It is intended to control local irritational factors.

D1120 prophylaxis – child

Removal of plaque, calculus and stains from the tooth structures in the primary and transitional dentition. It is intended to control local irritational factors.

a) Note localized inflammation. Generally healthy periodontium with no loss of attachment.

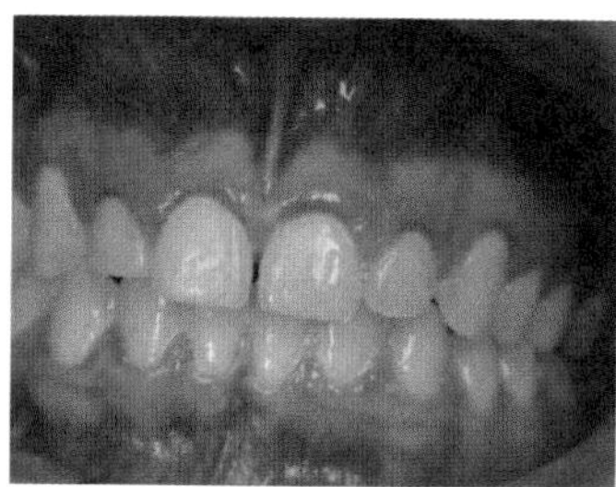

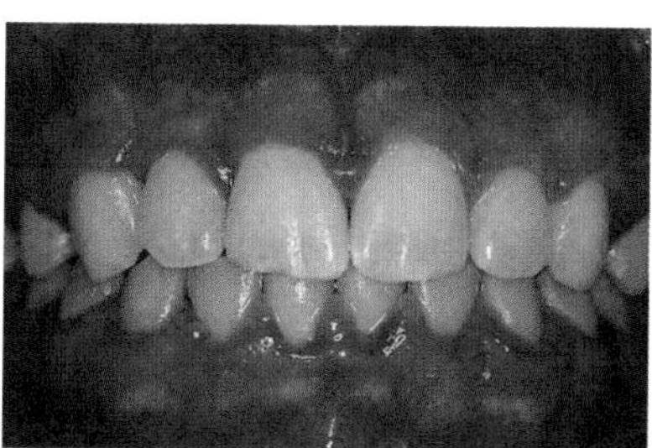

ADA American Dental Association®
America's leading advocate for oral health

b) Note stains and some supragingival deposits and localized inflammation but there is no bone loss.

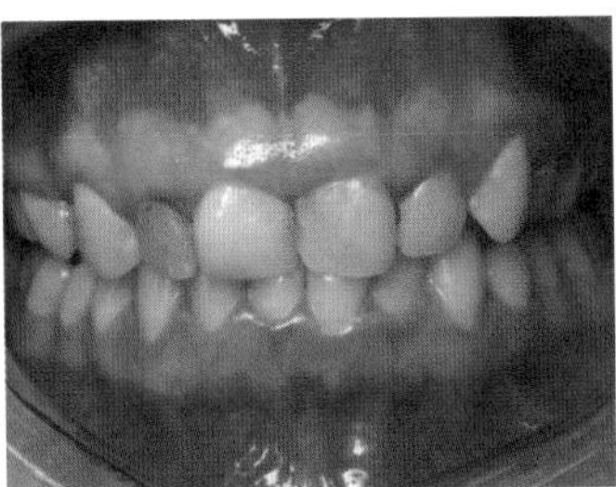

3. Illustrations of situation where scaling may be applicable

D4346 scaling in presence of generalized moderate or severe gingival inflammation – full mouth, after oral evaluation

The removal of plaque, calculus and stains from supra- and sub-gingival tooth surfaces when there is generalized moderate or severe gingival inflammation in the absence of periodontitis. It is indicated for patients who have swollen, inflamed gingiva, generalized suprabony pockets, and moderate to severe bleeding on probing. Should not be reported in conjunction with prophylaxis, scaling and root planing, or debridement procedures.

Note generalized inflammation with some pseudo-pockets. No apparent attachment loss.

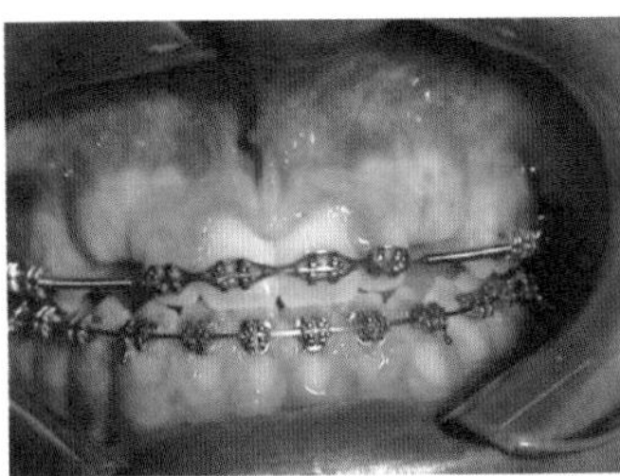

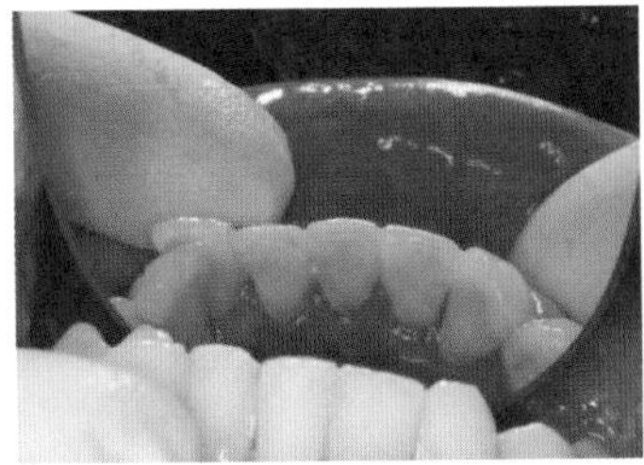

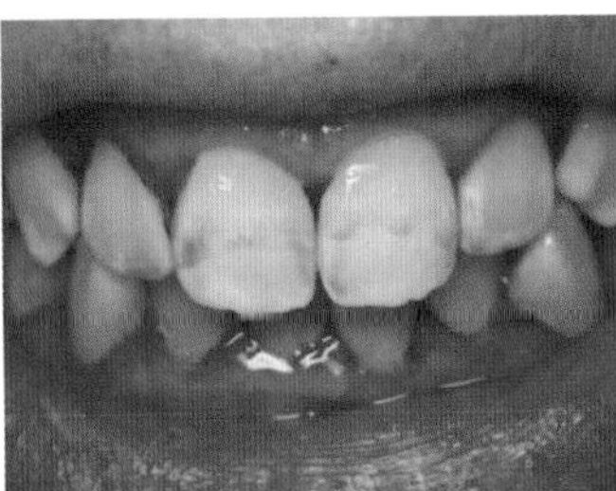

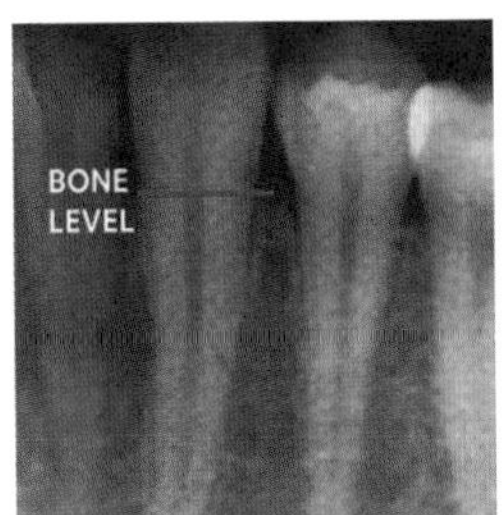

ADA American Dental Association®

America's leading advocate for oral health

D4346 Guide – Version 4 – July 11, 2018 – Page 10 of 11

4. Illustrations of situations for SRP and future periodontal maintenance

D4341 periodontal scaling and root planing – four or more teeth per quadrant

This procedure involves instrumentation of the crown and root surfaces of the teeth to remove plaque and calculus from these surfaces. It is indicated for patients with periodontal disease and is therapeutic, not prophylactic, in nature. Root planing is the definitive procedure designed for the removal of cementum and dentin that is rough, and/or permeated by calculus or contaminated with toxins or microorganisms. Some soft tissue removal occurs. This procedure may be used as a definitive treatment in some stages of periodontal disease and/or as a part of pre-surgical procedures in others.

D4342 periodontal scaling and root planing – one to three teeth per quadrant

This procedure involves instrumentation of the crown and root surfaces of the teeth to remove plaque and calculus from these surfaces. It is indicated for patients with periodontal disease and is therapeutic, not prophylactic, in nature. Root planing is the definitive procedure designed for the removal of cementum and dentin that is rough, and/or permeated by calculus or contaminated with toxins or microorganisms. Some soft tissue removal occurs. This procedure may be used as a definitive treatment in some stages of periodontal disease and/or as a part of pre-surgical procedures in others.

D4910 periodontal maintenance

This procedure is instituted following periodontal therapy and continues at varying intervals, determined by the clinical evaluation of the dentist, for the life of the dentition or any implant replacements. It includes removal of the bacterial plaque and calculus from supragingival and subgingival regions, site specific scaling and root planing where indicated, and polishing the teeth. If new or recurring periodontal disease appears, additional diagnostic and treatment procedures must be considered.

a) Photographic evidence of generalized attachment loss

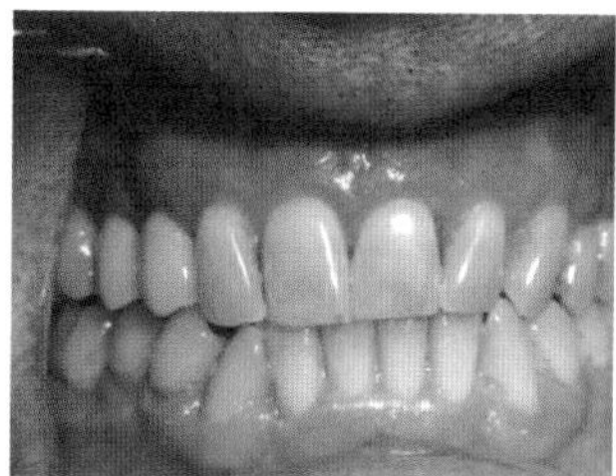

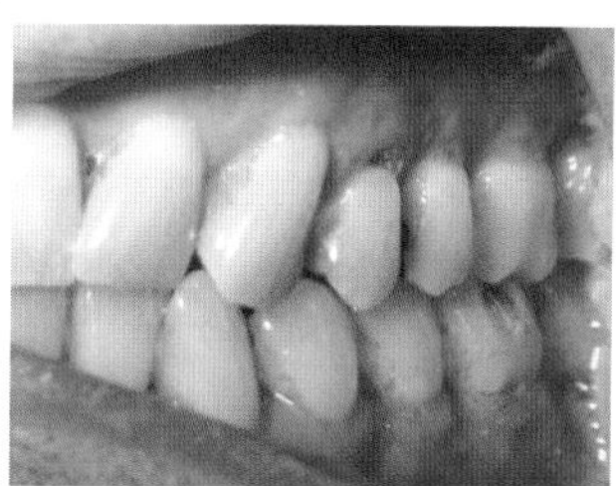

b) Radiographic evidence of bone loss

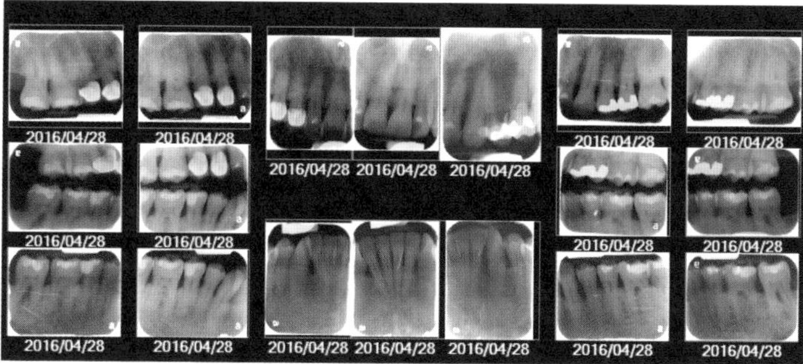

ADA American Dental Association®

America's leading advocate for oral health

c) Periodontal chart recording pocketing, attachment loss and bone loss

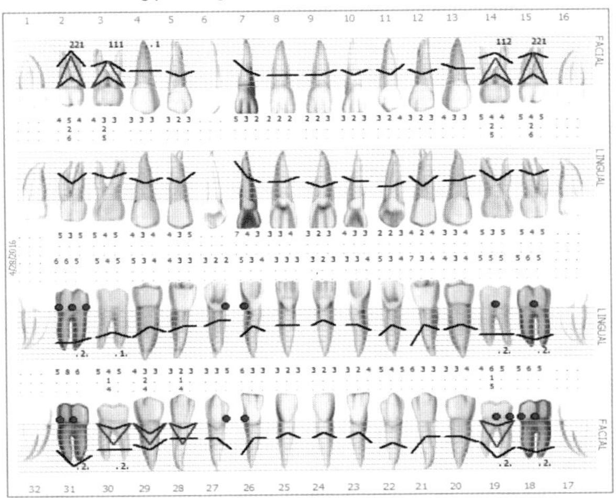

Questions or Assistance?

Call 800-621-8099 or send an email to dentalcode@ada.org

Notes:

-
- Version History

Date	Version	Remarks – Change Summary
05/16/2016	1	Initial publication
12/16/2016	2	Corrects answer 6.b) on page 3
		Adds Q&As 19-24 on page 6
10/25/2017	3	Editorial correction to question 15 on page 4 to remove obsolete reference to CDT 2017 in the question, and to simplify the answer for clarity; no change to the answer's original intent.
		Revises D4355 nomenclature and descriptor cited on page 7 to be consistent with the CDT 2018 revision
07/11/2018	4	Addition of new question, listed as #8, with following questions renumbered.

ADA American Dental Association®

America's leading advocate for oral health

Appendix 3: ADA Guide to Dental Procedures Reported with Area of the Oral Cavity or Tooth Anatomy (or Both)

This guide's focus is on claim submission completion – identifying by CDT code whether or not oral cavity area codes or tooth information should accompany the procedure code reported. It is also available online as a PDF at:

https://www.ada.org/en/publications/cdt/ada-dental-claim-form

ADA Dental Claim Data Content Recommendation - Reporting Area of the Oral Cavity and Tooth Anatomy by CDT Code - V2, Effective Jan 01, 2019

Dental procedure codes, listed in numeric order, are as published in CDT 2019 (© American Dental Association)

This recommendation:

1) Complements the ADA's compre http://www.ada.org/en/publications/cdt/ada-dental-claim-form
2) Is applicable to both the ADA Dental Claim Form (© 2012) and the HIPAA standard electronic dental claim transaction (837D v5010)

Notes:

a) For reference the Area of the Oral Cavity and the Tooth Anatomy code sets used on 837D and ADA Claim Form follow

Area of the Oral Cavity	entire oral cavity	00	upper right quadrant	10			
	maxillary arch	01	upper left quadrant	20			
	mandibular arch	02	lower left quadrant	30			
			lower right quadrant	40			
Tooth Anatomy	Number				Primary	Permanent	
		Maxillary (Patient Right to Left)			A - J	1 - 16	
		Mandibular (Patient Left to Right)			K - T	17 - 32	
	Surface	Mesial	M	Incisal	I	Facial (or Labial)	F
		Occlusal	O	Lingual	L		
		Distal	D	Buccal	B		

b) "X" in columns titled "N/R"= ADA does not recommend reporting any Area of the Oral Cavity or Tooth Anatomy information for that row's CDT code

c) "Y" in other columns under "Area of the Oral Cavity" or "Tooth Anatomy" = ADA recommends reporting the indicated information for that row's CDT code

Version History:

Number	Remarks / Change Summary	Date
1	Initial publication	Jan 2018
2	CDT 2019 update	Jan 2019

CDT Code	Area of the Oral Cavity				Tooth Anatomy			
#	N/R	Entire	Arch	Quadrant	N/R	#	# Range	Surface
D0120	X				X			
D0140	X				X			
D0145	X				X			
D0150	X				X			
D0160	X				X			
D0170	X				X			
D0171	X				X			
D0180	X				X			
D0190	X				X			
D0191	X				X			

ADA American Dental Association®
America's leading advocate for oral health

ADA Guide to Dental Procedures Reported with Area of the Oral Cavity or Tooth Anatomy (or Both)

Version 2 - January 2019

CDT Code	Area of the Oral Cavity				Tooth Anatomy			
#	N/R	Entire	Arch	Quadrant	N/R	#	# Range	Surface
D0210	X				X			
D0220	X					Y	Y	
D0230	X					Y	Y	
D0240	X						Y	
D0250	X						Y	
D0251	X						Y	
D0270	X						Y	
D0272	X						Y	
D0273	X						Y	
D0274	X						Y	
D0277	X						Y	
D0310	X				X			
D0320	X				X			
D0321	X				X			
D0322	X				X			
D0330		Y			X			
D0340	X				X			
D0350	X				X			
D0351	X				X			
D0364			X	X		X	X	
D0365	X				X			
D0366	X				X			
D0367	X				X			

ADA American Dental Association®
America's leading advocate for oral health

CDT Code	Area of the Oral Cavity				Tooth Anatomy			
#	N/R	Entire	Arch	Quadrant	N/R	#	# Range	Surface
D0368	X				X			
D0369	X				X			
D0370	X				X			
D0371	X				X			
D0380			X	X		X	X	
D0381	X				X			
D0382	X				X			
D0383	X				X			
D0384	X				X			
D0385	X				X			
D0386	X				X			
D0391	X				X			
D0393	X				X			
D0394	X				X			
D0395	X				X			
D0411	X				X			
D0412	X				X			
D0414	X				X			
D0415	X				X			
D0416	X				X			
D0417	X				X			
D0418	X				X			
D0422	X				X			

ADA Guide to Dental Procedures Reported with Area of the Oral Cavity or Tooth Anatomy (or Both)

Version 2 - January 2019

CDT Code	Area of the Oral Cavity				Tooth Anatomy			
#	N/R	Entire	Arch	Quadrant	N/R	#	# Range	Surface
D0423	X				X			
D0425	X				X			
D0431	X				X			
D0460	X					Y		
D0470	X	X			X			
D0472	X				X			
D0473	X				X			
D0474	X				X			
D0475	X				X			
D0476	X				X			
D0477	X				X			
D0478	X				X			
D0479	X				X			
D0480	X				X			
D0481	X				X			
D0482	X				X			
D0483	X				X			
D0484	X				X			
D0485	X				X			
D0486	X				X			
D0502	X				X			
D0600	X					Y	Y	
D0601	X				X			

ADA American Dental Association®
America's leading advocate for oral health

CDT Code	Area of the Oral Cavity				Tooth Anatomy			
#	N/R	Entire	Arch	Quadrant	N/R	#	# Range	Surface
D0602	X				X			
D0603	X				X			
D0999	X				X			
D1110		Y			X			
D1120		Y			X			
D1206		Y			X			
D1208		Y			X			
D1310	X				X			
D1320	X				X			
D1330	X				X			
D1351	X					Y		
D1352	X					Y		
D1353	X					Y		
D1354	X					Y		Y
D1510	X					Y	Y	
D1516	X					Y	Y	
D1517	X					Y	Y	
D1520	X					Y	Y	
D1526	X					Y	Y	
D1527	X					Y	Y	
D1550	X					Y	Y	
D1555	X					Y	Y	
D1575	X					Y	Y	

ADA American Dental Association®
America's leading advocate for oral health

ADA Guide to Dental Procedures Reported with Area of the Oral Cavity or Tooth Anatomy (or Both)

Version 2 - January 2019

CDT Code	Area of the Oral Cavity				Tooth Anatomy			
#	N/R	Entire	Arch	Quadrant	N/R	#	# Range	Surface
D1999				Y		Y	Y	
D2140	X					Y		Y
D2150	X					Y		Y
D2160	X					Y		Y
D2161	X					Y		Y
D2330	X					Y		Y
D2331	X					Y		Y
D2332	X					Y		Y
D2335	X					Y		Y
D2390	X					Y		
D2391	X					Y		Y
D2392	X					Y		Y
D2393	X					Y		Y
D2394	X					Y		Y
D2410	X					Y		Y
D2420	X					Y		Y
D2430	X					Y		Y
D2510	X					Y		Y
D2520	X					Y		Y
D2530	X					Y		Y
D2542	X					Y		Y
D2543	X					Y		Y
D2544	X					Y		Y

ADA American Dental Association®
America's leading advocate for oral health

CDT Code	Area of the Oral Cavity				Tooth Anatomy			
#	N/R	Entire	Arch	Quadrant	N/R	#	# Range	Surface
D2610	X					Y		Y
D2620	X					Y		Y
D2630	X					Y		Y
D2642	X					Y		Y
D2643	X					Y		Y
D2644	X					Y		Y
D2650	X					Y		Y
D2651	X					Y		Y
D2652	X					Y		Y
D2662	X					Y		Y
D2663	X					Y		Y
D2664	X					Y		Y
D2710	X					Y		
D2712	X					Y		
D2720	X					Y		
D2721	X					Y		
D2722	X					Y		
D2740	X					Y		
D2750	X					Y		
D2751	X					Y		
D2752	X					Y		
D2780	X					Y		
D2781	X					Y		

ADA American Dental Association®
America's leading advocate for oral health

ADA Guide to Dental Procedures Reported with Area of the Oral Cavity or Tooth Anatomy (or Both)

Version 2 - January 2019

CDT Code	Area of the Oral Cavity				Tooth Anatomy			
#	N/R	Entire	Arch	Quadrant	N/R	#	# Range	Surface
D2782	X					Y		
D2783	X					Y		
D2790	X					Y		
D2791	X					Y		
D2792	X					Y		
D2794	X					Y		
D2799	X					Y		
D2910	X					Y		
D2915	X					Y		
D2920	X					Y		
D2921	X					Y		
D2929	X					Y		
D2930	X					Y		
D2931	X					Y		
D2932	X					Y		
D2933	X					Y		
D2934	X					Y		
D2940	X					Y		Y
D2941	X					Y		Y
D2949	X					Y		Y
D2950	X					Y		
D2951	X					Y		
D2952	X					Y		

ADA American Dental Association®
America's leading advocate for oral health

CDT Code	Area of the Oral Cavity				Tooth Anatomy			
#	N/R	Entire	Arch	Quadrant	N/R	#	# Range	Surface
D2953	X					Y		
D2954	X					Y		
D2955	X					Y		
D2957	X					Y		
D2960	X					Y		
D2961	X					Y		
D2962	X					Y		
D2971	X					Y		
D2975	X					Y		
D2980	X					Y		
D2981	X					Y		
D2982	X					Y		
D2983	X					Y		
D2990	X					Y		Y
D2999	X					Y	Y	Y
D3110	X					Y		
D3120	X					Y		
D3220	X					Y		
D3221	X					Y		
D3222	X					Y		
D3230	X					Y		
D3240	X					Y		
D3310	X					Y		

ADA American Dental Association®
America's leading advocate for oral health

CDT Code	Area of the Oral Cavity				Tooth Anatomy			
#	N/R	Entire	Arch	Quadrant	N/R	#	# Range	Surface
D3320	X					Y		
D3330	X					Y		
D3331	X					Y		
D3332	X					Y		
D3333	X					Y		
D3346	X					Y		
D3347	X					Y		
D3348	X					Y		
D3351	X					Y		
D3352	X					Y		
D3353	X					Y		
D3355	X					Y		
D3356	X					Y		
D3357	X					Y		
D3410	X					Y		
D3421	X					Y		
D3425	X					Y		
D3426	X					Y		
D3427	X					Y		
D3428	X					Y		
D3429	X					Y		
D3430	X					Y		
D3431	X					Y		

ADA American Dental Association®
America's leading advocate for oral health

CDT Code	Area of the Oral Cavity				Tooth Anatomy			
#	N/R	Entire	Arch	Quadrant	N/R	#	# Range	Surface
D3432	X					Y		
D3450	X					Y		
D3460	X					Y		
D3470	X					Y		
D3910	X					Y		
D3920	X					Y		
D3950	X					Y		
D3999	X					Y	Y	
D4210				Y			Y	
D4211				Y			Y	
D4212	X					Y		
D4230				Y			Y	
D4231				Y			Y	
D4240				Y			Y	
D4241				Y			Y	
D4245	X						Y	
D4249	X					Y		
D4260				Y			Y	
D4261				Y			Y	
D4263				Y		Y		
D4264				Y		Y		
D4265	X					Y		
D4266	X					Y	Y	

ADA American Dental Association®
America's leading advocate for oral health

ADA Guide to Dental Procedures Reported with Area of the Oral Cavity or Tooth Anatomy (or Both)

Version 2 - January 2019

CDT Code	Area of the Oral Cavity				Tooth Anatomy			
#	N/R	Entire	Arch	Quadrant	N/R	#	# Range	Surface
D4267	X					Y	Y	
D4268	X					Y		
D4270	X					Y	Y	
D4273	X					Y		
D4274	X					Y		
D4275	X					Y		
D4276	X					Y		
D4277	X					Y		
D4278	X					Y		
D4283	X					Y		
D4285	X					Y		
D4320	X					Y		
D4321	X					Y		
D4341				Y		Y	Y	
D4342				Y		Y	Y	
D4346	X				X			
D4355	X				X			
D4381	X					Y		
D4910	X				X			
D4920	X					Y	Y	
D4921				Y	X			
D4999	X					Y	Y	
D5110	X				X			

ADA American Dental Association®
America's leading advocate for oral health

ADA Guide to Dental Procedures Reported with Area of the Oral Cavity or Tooth Anatomy (or Both)

CDT Code	Area of the Oral Cavity				Tooth Anatomy			
#	N/R	Entire	Arch	Quadrant	N/R	#	# Range	Surface
D5120	X				X			
D5130	X				X			
D5140	X				X			
D5211	X						Y	
D5212	X						Y	
D5213	X						Y	
D5214	X						Y	
D5221	X						Y	
D5222	X						Y	
D5223	X						Y	
D5224	X						Y	
D5225	X						Y	
D5226	X						Y	
D5282	X						Y	
D5283	X						Y	
D5410	X				X			
D5411	X				X			
D5421	X				X			
D5422	X				X			
D5511	X				X			
D5512	X				X			
D5520	X					Y		
D5611	X				X			

ADA American Dental Association®
America's leading advocate for oral health

ADA Guide to Dental Procedures Reported with Area of the Oral Cavity or Tooth Anatomy (or Both)

Version 2 - January 2019

CDT Code	Area of the Oral Cavity				Tooth Anatomy			
#	N/R	Entire	Arch	Quadrant	N/R	#	# Range	Surface
D5612	X				X			
D5621	X				X			
D5622	X				X			
D5630	X					Y		
D5640	X					Y		
D5650	X					Y		
D5660	X					Y		
D5670	X				X			
D5671	X				X			
D5710	X				X			
D5711	X				X			
D5720	X						Y	
D5721	X						Y	
D5730	X				X			
D5731	X				X			
D5740	X						Y	
D5741	X						Y	
D5750	X				X			
D5751	X				X			
D5760	X						Y	
D5761	X						Y	
D5810	X				X			
D5811	X				X			

ADA American Dental Association®
America's leading advocate for oral health

CDT Code	Area of the Oral Cavity				Tooth Anatomy			
#	N/R	Entire	Arch	Quadrant	N/R	#	# Range	Surface
D5820	X						Y	
D5821	X						Y	
D5850	X				X			
D5851	X				X			
D5862	X				X			
D5863	X				X			
D5864	X						Y	
D5865	X				X			
D5866	X						Y	
D5867				Y		Y	Y	
D5875			Y		X			
D5876			Y		X			
D5899	X					Y	Y	
D5911	X				X			
D5912	X				X			
D5913	X				X			
D5914	X				X			
D5915	X				X			
D5916	X				X			
D5919	X				X			
D5922	X				X			
D5923	X				X			
D5924	X				X			

ADA American Dental Association®
America's leading advocate for oral health

ADA Guide to Dental Procedures Reported with Area of the Oral Cavity or Tooth Anatomy (or Both)

Version 2 - January 2019

CDT Code	Area of the Oral Cavity				Tooth Anatomy			
#	N/R	Entire	Arch	Quadrant	N/R	#	# Range	Surface
D5925	X				X			
D5926	X				X			
D5927	X				X			
D5928	X				X			
D5929	X				X			
D5931			X		X			
D5932			X		X			
D5933			X		X			
D5934	X				X			
D5935	X				X			
D5936			Y		X			
D5937			Y		X			
D5951	X				X			
D5952			Y		X			
D5953			Y		X			
D5954	X				X			
D5955	X				X			
D5958	X				X			
D5959	X				X			
D5960			Y		X			
D5982			Y		X			
D5983			Y		X			
D5984			Y		X			

ADA American Dental Association®
America's leading advocate for oral health

CDT Code	Area of the Oral Cavity				Tooth Anatomy			
#	N/R	Entire	Arch	Quadrant	N/R	#	# Range	Surface
D5985			Y		X			
D5986			Y		X			
D5987			Y		X			
D5988			Y			Y		
D5991			Y		X			
D5992			Y		X			
D5993			Y		X			
D5994			Y			Y		
D5999	X				X			
D6010	X					Y		
D6011	X					Y		
D6012	X					Y		
D6013	X					Y		
D6040	X					Y		
D6050	X					Y		
D6051	X					Y		
D6052	X					Y		
D6055	X						Y	
D6056	X					Y		
D6057	X					Y		
D6058	X					Y		
D6059	X					Y		
D6060	X					Y		

ADA American Dental Association®
America's leading advocate for oral health

ADA Guide to Dental Procedures Reported with Area of the Oral Cavity or Tooth Anatomy (or Both)

Version 2 - January 2019

CDT Code	Area of the Oral Cavity				Tooth Anatomy			
#	N/R	Entire	Arch	Quadrant	N/R	#	# Range	Surface
D6061	X					Y		
D6062	X					Y		
D6063	X					Y		
D6064	X					Y		
D6065	X					Y		
D6066	X					Y		
D6067	X					Y		
D6068	X					Y		
D6069	X					Y		
D6070	X					Y		
D6071	X					Y		
D6072	X					Y		
D6073	X					Y		
D6074	X					Y		
D6075	X					Y		
D6076	X					Y		
D6077	X					Y		
D6080	X					Y		
D6081	X					Y		
D6085	X					Y		
D6090	X					Y		
D6091	X					Y		
D6092	X					Y		

ADA American Dental Association®
America's leading advocate for oral health

CDT Code	Area of the Oral Cavity				Tooth Anatomy			
#	N/R	Entire	Arch	Quadrant	N/R	#	# Range	Surface
D6093	X					Y		
D6094	X					Y		
D6095	X					Y		
D6096	X					Y		
D6100	X					Y		
D6101	X					Y		
D6102	X					Y		
D6103	X					Y	Y	
D6104	X					Y	Y	
D6110	X				X			
D6111	X				X			
D6112				Y	X			
D6113				Y	X			
D6114	X				X			
D6115	X				X			
D6116	X			Y	X			
D6117	X			Y	X			
D6118	X				X			
D6119	X				X			
D6190		Y		Y	X			
D6194	X				X			
D6199	X					Y	Y	
D6205	X					Y	Y	

ADA American Dental Association®
America's leading advocate for oral health

ADA Guide to Dental Procedures Reported with Area of the Oral Cavity or Tooth Anatomy (or Both)

Version 2 - January 2019

CDT Code	Area of the Oral Cavity				Tooth Anatomy			
#	N/R	Entire	Arch	Quadrant	N/R	#	# Range	Surface
D6210	X					Y	Y	
D6211	X					Y	Y	
D6212	X					Y	Y	
D6214	X					Y	Y	
D6240	X					Y	Y	
D6241	X					Y	Y	
D6242	X					Y	Y	
D6245	X					Y	Y	
D6250	X					Y	Y	
D6251	X					Y	Y	
D6252	X					Y	Y	
D6253	X					Y	Y	
D6545	X					Y		
D6548	X					Y		
D6549	X					Y		
D6600	X					Y		Y
D6601	X					Y		Y
D6602	X					Y		Y
D6603	X					Y		Y
D6604	X					Y		Y
D6605	X					Y		Y
D6606	X					Y		Y
D6607	X					Y		Y

ADA American Dental Association®
America's leading advocate for oral health

ADA Guide to Dental Procedures Reported with Area of the Oral Cavity or Tooth Anatomy (or Both)

CDT Code	Area of the Oral Cavity				Tooth Anatomy			
#	N/R	Entire	Arch	Quadrant	N/R	#	# Range	Surface
D6608	X					Y		Y
D6609	X					Y		Y
D6610	X					Y		Y
D6611	X					Y		Y
D6612	X					Y		Y
D6613	X					Y		Y
D6614	X					Y		Y
D6615	X					Y		Y
D6624	X					Y		
D6634	X					Y		
D6710	X					Y		
D6720	X					Y		
D6721	X					Y		
D6722	X					Y		
D6740	X					Y		
D6750	X					Y		
D6751	X					Y		
D6752	X					Y		
D6780	X					Y		
D6781	X					Y		
D6782	X					Y		
D6783	X					Y		
D6790	X					Y		

ADA American Dental Association®
America's leading advocate for oral health

ADA Guide to Dental Procedures Reported with Area of the Oral Cavity or Tooth Anatomy (or Both)

Version 2 - January 2019

CDT Code	Area of the Oral Cavity				Tooth Anatomy			
#	N/R	Entire	Arch	Quadrant	N/R	#	# Range	Surface
D6791	X					Y		
D6792	X					Y		
D6793	X					Y		
D6794	X					Y		
D6920			Y				Y	
D6930	X				X			
D6940	X					Y		Y
D6950	X					Y		
D6980	X				X			
D6985			Y	Y	X			
D6999			Y	Y		Y	Y	Y
D7111	X					Y		
D7140	X					Y		
D7210	X					Y		
D7220	X					Y		
D7230	X					Y		
D7240	X					Y		
D7241	X					Y		
D7250	X					Y		
D7251	X					Y		
D7260				Y	X			
D7261				Y	X			
D7270	X				X			

ADA American Dental Association®
America's leading advocate for oral health

CDT Code	Area of the Oral Cavity				Tooth Anatomy			
#	N/R	Entire	Arch	Quadrant	N/R	#	# Range	Surface
D7272	X				X			
D7280	X					Y		
D7282	X					Y		
D7283	X					Y		
D7285		Y			X			
D7286		Y			X			
D7287		Y			X			
D7288		Y			X			
D7290	X				X			
D7291	X				X			
D7292				Y	X			
D7293				Y	X			
D7294				Y	X			
D7295				Y	X			
D7296				Y		Y	Y	
D7297				Y		Y	Y	
D7310				Y		Y	Y	
D7311				Y		Y	Y	
D7320				Y		Y	Y	
D7321				Y		Y	Y	
D7340				Y	X			
D7350				Y	X			
D7410			X		X			

ADA American Dental Association®
America's leading advocate for oral health

ADA Guide to Dental Procedures Reported with Area of the Oral Cavity or Tooth Anatomy (or Both)

Version 2 - January 2019

CDT Code	Area of the Oral Cavity				Tooth Anatomy			
#	N/R	Entire	Arch	Quadrant	N/R	#	# Range	Surface
D7411			X		X			
D7412			X		X			
D7413			X		X			
D7414			X		X			
D7415			X		X			
D7440			X		X			
D7441			X		X			
D7450			X		X			
D7451			X		X			
D7460			X		X			
D7461			X		X			
D7465			X		X			
D7471			Y		X			
D7472	X				X			
D7473				Y	X			
D7485				Y	X			
D7490			Y		X			
D7510				Y		Y		
D7511				Y		Y		
D7520			Y		X			
D7521			Y		X			
D7530	X				X			
D7540	X				X			

ADA American Dental Association®

America's leading advocate for oral health

CDT Code	Area of the Oral Cavity				Tooth Anatomy			
#	N/R	Entire	Arch	Quadrant	N/R	#	# Range	Surface
D7550				Y	X			
D7560	X				X			
D7610	X				X			
D7620	X				X			
D7630	X				X			
D7640	X				X			
D7650	X				X			
D7660	X				X			
D7670	X				X			
D7671	X				X			
D7680	X				X			
D7710	X				X			
D7720	X				X			
D7730	X				X			
D7740	X				X			
D7750	X				X			
D7760	X				X			
D7770	X				X			
D7771	X				X			
D7780	X				X			
D7010	X				X			
D7820	X				X			
D7830	X				X			

ADA American Dental Association®
America's leading advocate for oral health

ADA Guide to Dental Procedures Reported with Area of the Oral Cavity or Tooth Anatomy (or Both)

Version 2 - January 2019

CDT Code	Area of the Oral Cavity				Tooth Anatomy			
#	N/R	Entire	Arch	Quadrant	N/R	#	# Range	Surface
D7840	X				X			
D7850	X				X			
D7852	X				X			
D7854	X				X			
D7856	X				X			
D7858	X				X			
D7860	X				X			
D7865	X				X			
D7870	X				X			
D7871	X				X			
D7872	X				X			
D7873	X				X			
D7874	X				X			
D7875	X				X			
D7876	X				X			
D7877	X				X			
D7880	X				X			
D7881	X				X			
D7899	X				X			
D7910	X				X			
D7911	X				X			
D7912	X				X			
D7920	X				X			

ADA American Dental Association®

America's leading advocate for oral health

CDT Code	Area of the Oral Cavity				Tooth Anatomy			
#	N/R	Entire	Arch	Quadrant	N/R	#	# Range	Surface
D7921	X				X			
D7940	X				X			
D7941	X				X			
D7943	X				X			
D7944	X				X			
D7945	X				X			
D7946	X				X			
D7947	X				X			
D7948	X				X			
D7949	X				X			
D7950	X				X			
D7951	X				X			
D7952	X				X			
D7953	X				X			
D7955	X				X			
D7960	X				X			
D7963	X				X			
D7970			Y		X			
D7971	X				X			
D7972				Y	X			
D7979	X				X			
D7980	X				X			
D7981	X				X			

ADA Guide to Dental Procedures Reported with Area of the Oral Cavity or Tooth Anatomy (or Both)

CDT Code	Area of the Oral Cavity				Tooth Anatomy			
#	N/R	Entire	Arch	Quadrant	N/R	#	# Range	Surface
D7982	X				X			
D7983	X				X			
D7990	X				X			
D7991	X				X			
D7995	X				X			
D7996	X				X			
D7997			X		X			
D7998	X				X			
D7999	X				X			
D8010			Y	Y	X			
D8020			Y	Y	X			
D8030			Y	Y	X			
D8040			Y	Y	X			
D8050		Y	Y	Y	X			
D8060		Y	Y	Y	X			
D8070		Y			X			
D8080		Y			X			
D8090		Y			X			
D8210		Y	Y	Y	X			
D8220		Y	Y	Y	X			
D8660		Y			X			
D8670		Y			X			
D8680		Y	Y	Y	X			

ADA American Dental Association®
America's leading advocate for oral health

CDT Code	Area of the Oral Cavity				Tooth Anatomy			
#	N/R	Entire	Arch	Quadrant	N/R	#	# Range	Surface
D8681			Y		X			
D8690		Y	Y	Y	X			
D8691		Y	Y	Y	X			
D8692		Y	Y	Y	X			
D8693		Y	Y	Y	X			
D8694		Y	Y	Y	X			
D8695		Y	Y	Y	X			
D8999	X				X			
D9110	X				X			
D9120	X				X			
D9130	X				X			
D9210			Y	Y	X			
D9211			Y	Y	X			
D9212			Y	Y	X			
D9215			Y	Y	X			
D9219	X				X			
D9222	X				X			
D9223	X				X			
D9230	X				X			
D9239	X				X			
D9243	X				Y			
D9248	X				X			
D9310	X				X			

ADA American Dental Association®
America's leading advocate for oral health

ADA Guide to Dental Procedures Reported with Area of the Oral Cavity or Tooth Anatomy (or Both)

Version 2 - January 2019

CDT Code	Area of the Oral Cavity				Tooth Anatomy			
#	N/R	Entire	Arch	Quadrant	N/R	#	# Range	Surface
D9311	X				X			
D9410	X				X			
D9420	X				X			
D9430	X				X			
D9440	X				X			
D9450	X				X			
D9610	X				X			
D9612	X				X			
D9613	X				X			
D9630	X				X			
D9910			Y	Y	X			
D9911	X					Y		
D9920	X				X			
D9930	X				X			
D9932	X				X			
D9933	X				X			
D9934	X				X			
D9935	X				X			
D9944			Y		X			
D9945			Y		X			
D9946			Y		X			
D9941			Y		X			
D9942			Y		X			

ADA American Dental Association®

America's leading advocate for oral health

CDT Code	Area of the Oral Cavity				Tooth Anatomy			
#	N/R	Entire	Arch	Quadrant	N/R	#	# Range	Surface
D9943			Y		X			
D9950			Y		X			
D9951			Y	Y	X			
D9952			Y	Y	X			
D9961	X				X			
D9970	X				X			
D9971	X					Y	Y	
D9972			Y		X			
D9973	X					Y		
D9974	X					Y		
D9975			Y		X			
D9985	X				X			
D9986	X				X			
D9987	X				X			
D9990	X				X			
D9991	X				X			
D9992	X				X			
D9993	X				X			
D9994	X				X			
D9995	X				X			
D9996	X				X			
D9999	X				X			

ADA American Dental Association®
America's leading advocate for oral health